A STEP-BY-STEP GUIDE

HEAD, NECK & SHOULDERS MASSAGE

A STEP-BY-STEP GUIDE

HEAD, NECK & SHOULDERS MASSAGE

EILEAN BENTLEY

St. Martin's Griffin New York

A Gaia original

Books from Gaia celebrate the vision of Gaia, the self-sustaining living Earth, and seek to help its readers live in greater personal and planetary harmony.

Editors	Katherine Pate, Sarah Townsend
Designer	Mark Epton
Art Director	Lucy Guenot
Photographer	Steve Teague
Managing Editor	Pip Morgan
Production	Lyn Kirby
Direction	Joss Pearson, Patrick Nugent

ISBN 0-312-24720-6

First published in the United Kingdom by Gaia Books Limited. First US edition: September 2000.

10 9 8 7 6 5 4 3 2 1

Note on safety

The techniques and treatments in this book are to be used at the reader's sole discretion and risk. Always observe the cautions and consult a doctor if you are in any doubt about a medical condition.

About this book

This step-by-step guide shows you how to use a unique combination of head massage, and meditations or visualizations, to promote health and wellbeing in mind, body, and spirit.

The introduction explains how the massage and meditation techniques combine to form a truly holistic therapy, working with the body's life force, or energy.

Chapter one presents the basic techniques, while chapter two explains how to use meditation and visualization. These are then combined in a self-care routine in chapter three.

Chapter four focuses on using meditation to develop the senses, and chapter five presents the complete massage plan.

Regular head massage following the routines in chapters three and five has many health benefits. In addition, chapter six gives techniques to treat 25 common ailments and conditions.

Cautions

Head massage is very safe, but some people should be treated with care. Cautions relating to specific steps of the massage are explained in the step-by-step treatments. Please also observe the following.

The very young, the elderly, and those suffering from bone problems
Use light massage only. Pressure should not exceed the weight of your fingers: even the weight of your hand can be excessive.

Sufferers of epilepsy and clinical depression
The top of the head is a particularly sensitive area for these conditions. Use light massage only, no more than stroking and combing with your fingers.

Pregnant women
Head massage can be of great benefit during pregnancy but some special care is needed. Follow the guidelines given on page 127 in chapter six.

Cancer sufferers
Those being treated for any form of cancer, and those in remission, need extra care. A light head massage treatment will be of great benefit, but as the lymphatic system can transfer some forms of cancer to other parts of the body, avoid working on the lymphatic areas illustrated on page 107.

Sufferers of low blood pressure
Head massage lowers the blood pressure, so anyone who already has low blood pressure should have only a light treatment lasting no longer than 15 minutes.

Contents

Introduction

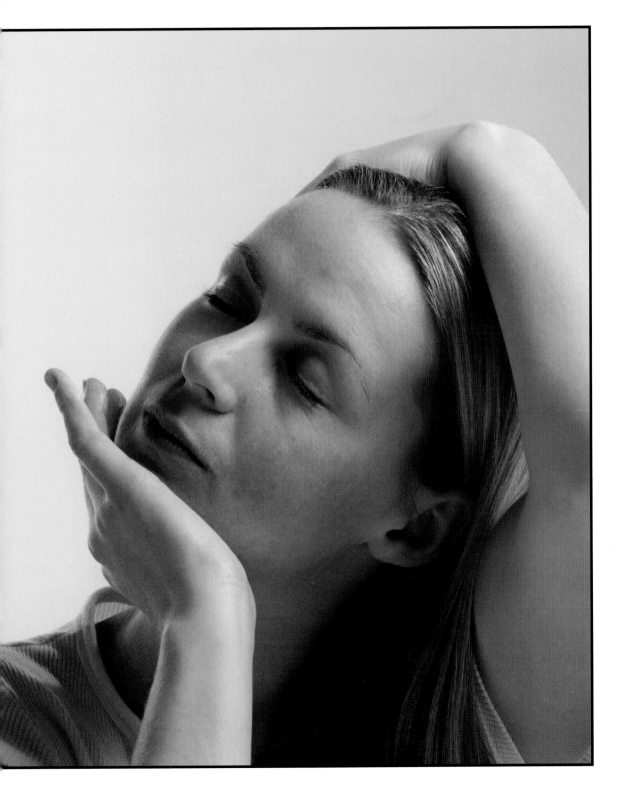

Introduction

Good health depends on balanced energy. This energy, called chi or ki in Oriental medicine, or prana in Indian tradition, is the life force itself. It permeates our bodies and every living thing in the universe. When our energy is unbalanced we may feel mildly irritable, out of sorts, or even seriously unwell.

Stress, poor diet, strong emotions, or toxin build-up are all symptoms of modern living that can unbalance life energy and create areas of negativity. The power of energy healing lies in rebalancing the life force so that the flow of energy within us is constant, effortless, and unblocked. Head massage, combined with simple meditative techniques, provides a simple and effective way to rebalance our energies and clear any areas of negativity, easing and even preventing many illnesses.

Many of the head massage techniques in this book are based on traditional Indian head massage. Some are drawn from other ancient and traditional methods of healing such as shiatsu, reiki, acupressure, and qi gong. Although each uses different terminology to explain the theory, they are all based on a common concept. Life energy flows within us and, by working on the channels it flows through, or specific points or areas, this energy can be brought into balance.

Head massage also affects the pulsing rhythms of cerebrospinal fluid, carrying healing messages around the body and stimulating the body's self-healing mechanisms. Tension in the muscles is released, dispersing toxins, reducing mental and physical stress, and improving blood flow to the brain.

Sharing head massage

You can use any head massage strokes on yourself, and a self-care routine is introduced in chapter three. However, the treatment is much more effective if someone else massages you, as they can talk you through the meditations or visualizations, while you relax and let go completely. Sharing the experience with a friend or partner, and taking turns to give a massage, greatly enhances the healing qualities of the techniques. You will both benefit as much from the giving as the receiving.

Touch alone is very powerful, but another vital ingredient in head massage is the intention of the giver to transmit healing, caring, love, and wellbeing to the receiver. The meditations and visualizations that accompany the massage techniques help here: by centering and grounding the giver, and channeling the feelings and emotions, they allow the receiver to take an active part in their own healing.

Meditations and visualizations allow you to tap into the universal healing energy and transmit this to your partner. By calming the mind, meditation allows this energy to flow freely. Visualization enables you to direct it to specific areas where it is needed, either within your body or in your aura – the energy field surrounding your physical body. Many illnesses originate in energy disturbances in the aura, so using visualization to cleanse it is an effective preventive treatment. The combination of massage and meditation is a truly holistic therapy that benefits the entire mental, emotional, spiritual, and physical being.

This book is not just about giving and receiving a relaxing massage. It is about the energies of two people becoming completely as one, for the benefit of the healing process.

Positions for treatment

Traditional Indian head massage is usually given with
the receiver seated. However, some people prefer to be
massaged lying down. You should choose whichever feels
more comfortable for you and your partner.

With your partner sitting it is very easy to reach all areas of
the head, neck, and shoulders. However this position may not
be ideal for really deep massage. The more relaxed your
partner becomes, the more she will slump in the chair, which
can become rather uncomfortable for both of you. Only light,
simple meditations can be used, such as asking your partner
to focus on rippling waves or color changes in a crystal.

For a deep, relaxing massage it may be better for your partner
to lie on her back on the floor, on some padding such as an
exercise mat, or a couple of duvets. In this position the body
can enter a state of deep relaxation, allowing its own healing
mechanisms to work. Now you can use a strong meditation or
visualization as part of the treatment, such as floating down a
river or flying through clouds, to help with the healing process.

However, it is more difficult to reach areas on the back of the
head and neck with your partner lying down, and you will
often have to turn the head to the side and support it with
your hand. You will need to kneel or sit behind your partner's
head, and may have to move around to reach different areas.

Whichever position your partner chooses, you need to be
relaxed and comfortable yourself in order to guide her into
deep relaxation. Wear loose fitting clothing so you can move
around easily, especially if you are working on the floor. If you
need to change position during the treatment, move slowly
and rhythmically so your partner is unaware of any break.

To work with your partner seated, select a chair that is high
enough for you to reach the scalp and shoulders without
bending. Your partner should sit with feet flat on the floor,
hands in her lap, and shoulders back. Stand squarely behind
her. You should wear comfortable shoes or have bare feet,
and maintain a straight posture.

Creating a soothing atmosphere

Before starting a treatment you should prepare yourself and your surroundings. The room should be comfortably warm, but not stuffy. Lower the lighting or use candles, and burn incense or oil. It is a good idea to check first if your partner has any preferences, as smells have very different associations for different individuals. Some suggestions are given in the box below. Some people like to play soothing music, others prefer silence. Choose whatever feels best for you and your partner.

If it is not possible to burn oils or play music, perhaps at the office, you can still prepare the space by clearing away any clutter and making sure you will not be interrupted while you are massaging your partner.

Essential oils	
Lavender	lifts the spirits
Sandalwood	relieves stress and lifts the spirits
White pine	creates a feeling of space and openness
Geranium	lifts the mood
Eucalyptus	treats the first symptoms of cold and respiratory problems
Frankincense	relaxes, uplifts, relieves depression, and creates a feeling of sacred space
Citrus	clears the head and lifts the spirits

Cleansing visualizations

Before you begin to massage your partner, you can perform this simple visualization to cleanse the energy of the space in which you are working.

Sit for a few moments in the middle of the space. Close your eyes and visualize a gold ring spinning just above your head. Watch it growing larger and descending so that it comes down around your body, leaving behind a golden trace as it descends, enveloping you in a bubble. Watch the energy within this bubble turn to a soft pink, and move this energy outward from you until it fills the whole space or room.

You have now surrounded yourself in a protective energy field, which will stop any negative energy from your partner reaching you, and vice versa. You have created a healing space filled with this protective energy.

At the end of your massage session, after you have broken contact with your partner, use this visualization to clear your energy and the energy of the space.

Sit for a few moments and again visualize the space filled with pink, healing energy. Slowly bring the bubble in around you. See the gold ring spinning beneath you. Move the ring up around your body until it is above your head. Feel the energy rising up through your body with the gold ring. Then watch the ring grow smaller and slowly rise up out of sight.

Making and breaking the energy connection

Before any massage session with a partner you should make an energy connection between you. This enables you to tap into the healing energy of the universe and allow it to channel through you into your partner, maximizing the healing power of the treatment. It also synchronizes you both, allowing you to understand your partner's needs instinctively.

At the end of a treatment it is equally important to break the connection between you. This allows you both to take back complete control of your own energy flow, as well as sending any negative energy back into the universe to be cleansed. No links will remain that could drain your energy or your partner's. This may seem a strange concept, but the more sensitive you become to the flowing of energy, the more you will appreciate its movements, directions, and strengths.

Full instructions for making and breaking the energy connection are given in the massage plans.

After a treatment, you should allow time for your partner to come back to reality. A deeply relaxing massage can leave the recipient feeling a little light-headed. Spend some time chatting quietly and have a cup of tea or other non-alcoholic drink until you both feel more grounded.

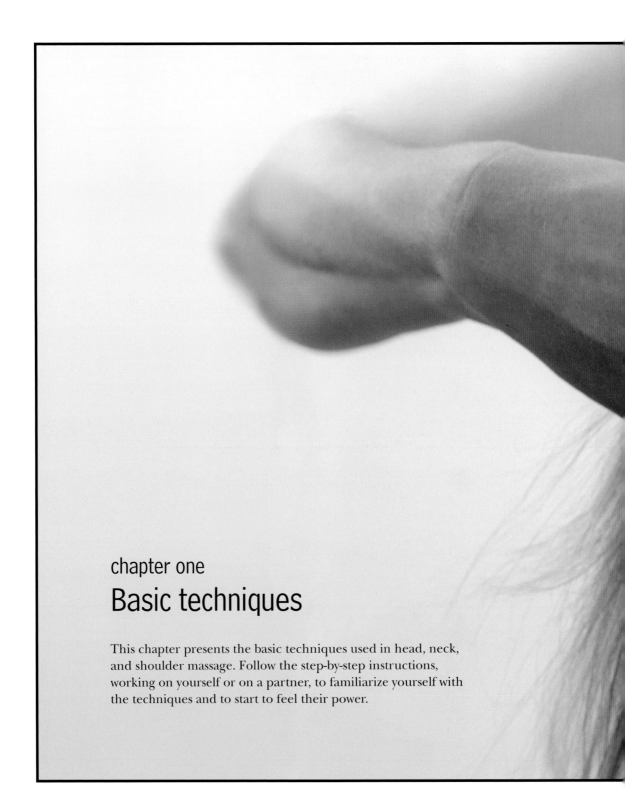

chapter one
Basic techniques

This chapter presents the basic techniques used in head, neck, and shoulder massage. Follow the step-by-step instructions, working on yourself or on a partner, to familiarize yourself with the techniques and to start to feel their power.

Basic techniques

The position of points and areas to massage are often described using fingerwidths; for example, "massage along the jawbone at two fingerwidth intervals". Because parts of the body are in proportion, and someone with small hands will usually also have a small overall bone structure, using your massage partner's personal fingerwidth measurement helps you locate the correct areas on that person. So before you start to give a massage, look at the width of your partner's index finger and use that measurement when necessary.

Always use both hands in massage. If you are working with one hand only, use the other to support your partner. This maintains and strengthens the contact between you, and helps to relax your partner and hold him in position.

For all the techniques in this chapter – unless specified otherwise – sit your partner in a chair and stand squarely behind him. Most of the movements described require you to work in regular lines over the head and upper body (see illustration opposite). This is reassuring for your partner, as he then knows where to expect the next touch. It also helps to ensure that you cover the whole area effectively.

When you have finished using one technique, stroke or gently comb through your partner's hair with your fingers. This relaxing and soothing action loosens the hair ready for the next treatment. If you have been supporting your partner's head with your hand, it also allows him to take control of his head again before you move to a new position.

Let your partner guide you on how much pressure to use. Too light a pressure can be irritating, but the massage should not cause discomfort.

Caution
Do not use firm pressure on the top of the head on the very young, the elderly, or anyone suffering from epilepsy, bone disease, or clinical depression. Also observe the cautions on page 5.

Rotations

This technique should be used in a slow, meditative way. You can use one or more fingers, your thumbs, the heel of your hand, or your whole hand. Work in regular lines over your partner (see below, right) to help him relax and enjoy the experience.

These movements stimulate the circulation, move stagnant blood and energy, and tone and loosen the muscles. Rotations on the head also stimulate the scalp and improve hair condition.

One finger rotations
Cup your right hand on the forehead, taking care not to push down on the eyebrows. Place the pad of the index or middle finger of your left hand in the centre of the forehead at the hairline. Using firm pressure, rotate your finger for three to five seconds. Then move two fingerwidths back along the midline and repeat the rotation. Continue until you reach the nape of the neck.

Working in lines
Now place your finger on the hairline two fingerwidths to the left of your first line. Work back in a line parallel to the first, ending at the nape of the neck. Continue to work lines back over the head until you have covered the left half, finishing with a line running just above the ear. Stroke the hair gently with both hands, then use your right hand to work back in lines on the right side of the head.

19

Rotations

Rotations with two or more fingers

Using two or more fingers reduces the amount of pressure you exert, while allowing you to cover a greater area. Start with your fingers about 1cm (½in) apart on the hairline, and work back over the head in lines as for one finger rotations.

If you start in the middle of the hairline with all four fingers you will be able to cover the top of the head down to the nape of the neck in one sweep. You can then use the four fingers of both hands, one either side of the head, to work both sides of the head together.

Thumb rotations: back

This technique is used on the upper back, shoulders, and neck, but not on the head as it exerts strong pressure. To increase the pressure further, lean into your thumbs as you work.

Place the pads of your thumbs either side of the spine, level with the base of the shoulder blades and rotate firmly for three to five seconds. Then move your thumbs two fingerwidths outward in a horizontal line and rotate again. Repeat, moving two fingerwidths along this line each time, until you reach the edges of the back.

Now start either side of the spine again, two fingerwidths up from your first line, and work a parallel line. Repeat until you reach the neck.

Caution
Do not apply strong pressure directly on the spine.

Thumb rotations: neck

Rest your fingers on the shoulders and use thumb rotations in horizontal lines from each side of the spine outward until you reach the base of the skull.

Caution
Do not massage this part of the neck on anyone who has cancer.

Heel of hand rotations: back

This technique uses firm pressure over a larger area than the thumb rotations. To increase the pressure, lean into your hands as you work. Start with the heels of your hands on either side of the spine, level with the lower edge of the shoulder blades. Rotate, using strong pressure and small movements. Then move two fingerwidths outward on a horizontal line and repeat. Continue out to the edges and then in parallel lines up the back, as for thumb rotations.

Increasing the pressure

For stronger pressure, brace your partner with your arm across the front of the shoulders and use one hand to work parallel lines over one half of the back. Change hands and repeat on the other side.

Heel of hand rotations: head

Support the forehead carefully with one hand, place the heel of your hand at the nape of the neck and rotate using small, gentle movements. Work a line up the middle of the head and over the top to the forehead.

This movement can also be used on the sides of the head, working in lines from the back of the head to the front (see rotations with two or more fingers, page 20).

Whole hand rotations

To apply a lighter pressure over a larger area, use the whole hand, following the movements for heel of hand rotations.

Pressure

For this technique you can use your fingers, thumbs, hands, or elbows, and lean in with your body weight to vary the amount of pressure used. When working on very tense areas of your partner's body, a continuous whole-body rocking action of pressure and release is very effective. Alternatively, keep the massage quiet and still, holding the pressure for three to five seconds before moving to the next point.

This technique loosens tension and stiffness in muscles and is particularly effective in treating stress and tension headaches. It also balances and boosts energy levels, and subtly corrects pressure imbalances in the cerebrospinal fluid.

Thumb pressure
Use thumbs together or separately to apply pressure to the upper back, shoulders, and neck. Before exerting strong pressure, ask your partner to brace herself by pressing her hands against her knees.
Start with your thumbs either side of the spine, level with the bottom of the shoulder blades. Lean forward, with your weight on your thumbs, hold for three to five seconds, then release. Work outward from the spine in parallel horizontal lines up the back. At the base of the neck, use your thumbs on either side of the spine. Press upward for three to five seconds, release, and move two fingerwidths to the next point. Continue until you reach the nape of the neck.
Alternatively, work with one thumb, supporting your partner with your other arm across the front of the shoulders. Work across one half of the back from the spine outward and give the back a vigorous rub before changing hands and working on the other side.

Caution
Do not massage this part of the neck on anyone who has cancer.

Finger pressure
Support the head with your left hand. Starting in the middle of the hairline, use one or more fingers to apply a firm pressure for three to five seconds, then release. Cover one half of the head, working back in parallel lines to the nape of the neck, then change hands and work over the other half.

Heel of hand pressure

This technique applies less intense pressure over a larger area, and is more comfortable for very tender areas. You can use it on the back, neck, shoulders, and back of the head. Support your partner with one arm across the front of her shoulders and lean your weight slowly onto the heel of the other hand. Gently increase the pressure outward from the spine, across the back as before and moving up in lines until you reach the neck. Change hands and work on the other half of the back, then give the whole area a vigorously rub.

To use this technique on the back of the head, support your partner's forehead with one hand.

Elbow pressure

Strong pressure from the elbows is good for releasing tension in the shoulders. Standing behind your partner, place your elbows on the tops of her shoulders, close to the base of the neck. Then raise your hands back toward you, leaning your body weight onto the shoulders. Hold for three to five seconds, then release the pressure, dropping your hands forward again. Repeat at four fingerwidth intervals along the shoulders until you reach the tops of the arms.

Caution

Do not massage the midpoint of the shoulders of anyone who is pregnant.

Forearm pressure

This technique can be used to release tension in the shoulders if the area is tender. With your hands held in loose fists, rest the backs of your forearms on the tops of the shoulders, close to the base of the neck. Lean down firmly and hold for three to five seconds, then rock your body back to release. Repeat at four fingerwidth intervals along the tops of the shoulders.

Rolling

This technique is used on the head, neck, and shoulders. Use the outside edge of the hands, rolling along the line of the little fingers with a constant flowing rhythm.

Rolling relaxes mind and body, tones the scalp, and helps to ease tension.

Using both hands together enables you to work on both sides of the head simultaneously. With your fingers straight, use the outside edge of the heels of your hands to make contact with the sides of the head. Now roll the pressure up the edges of your hands to the tips of your little fingers. Roll back down to the heels of the hands, maintaining a smooth rhythm. Move two fingerwidths up the head each time, following parallel lines, to cover the whole area.
For a stronger treatment, roll with one hand at a time, supporting the head with the other.

Knuckling

This technique uses the knuckles on the head, neck, and shoulders. For less pressure you can use the top set of knuckles, just below the fingernails.

This is a vigorous and stimulating treatment, which boosts energy levels and encourages deeper breathing.

Curl your hands into fists and rest them on the shoulders. Rock the fists from side to side, from the little finger to the index finger and back again. The pressure should be firm and steady. Move slowly all over the head and shoulders, following parallel lines. On the neck, start next to the spine and work outward in parallel lines moving up to the nape.

Caution
Do not massage the midpoint of the shoulders of anyone who is pregnant.

Pulling

In these techniques the hair is pulled slowly and evenly, without tweaking, to stimulate the muscles under the scalp.

Pulling releases tension in these muscles and can be used to treat tension headaches. It also conditions the hair by stimulating blood flow to the scalp.

Lying down

Start at the front of the head. Turn your hands so the palms face outward, and push your fingers through the hair from the temples. Grip the hair firmly between your fingers and pull steadily and firmly.

Sitting down

Start by combing your fingers lightly through the hair to loosen it. With your hands on either side of the neck, slide them up into the hair, fingers apart, keeping close to the scalp. When you have gathered a handful of hair, close your fingers firmly and pull away from the head. Allow the hair to move through your fingers under tension, creating a strong, even pull. Repeat all over the head, always pulling the hair at right angles away from the scalp.

Twisting and pulling

Starting in the middle of the hairline, wrap a small section of hair around your finger and hold firmly for three to five seconds. Release and repeat two fingerwidths back along the midline to the nape of the neck. Return to the hairline and work in parallel lines to cover each side of the head in turn. Run your fingers up through the hair from the nape of the neck to the front of the head, to ease out the scalp.

Kneading

Use finger or thumb kneading on the head or face, or knead with the heel of your hand or lightly clenched fist on the head, neck, back, and shoulders.

Kneading is a wonderfully stimulating and energizing massage technique.

Heel of hand kneading
Support the forehead carefully with one hand. Place the heel of the other hand at the nape of the neck, applying pressure while rolling from the heel up over the palm to the fingertips. Work up to the front of the head along the midline. Then work up the sides in the same way, starting at the nape each time.

Finger kneading
Support the head with your left hand. Using the middle finger of your right hand to press on your right index finger, start in the middle of the hairline and work back along the midline at two fingerwidth intervals. Knead in parallel lines over the sides of the head. For stronger pressure, use the thumb for kneading.

Clenched fist kneading
Clench your hand loosely into a fist, and press as you roll up from the heel of your hand to the knuckles. Work up the head in the same way as for heel of hand kneading.

Scratching

For this technique, used on the head, nails need to be short to avoid snagging your partner's scalp.

Scratching stimulates blood flow to the scalp, improving the flow of nutrients to the hair roots.

Hold your hands with your fingers together and bent so that your nails are in line. This reduces the strength you can exert and lessens the chance of catching your partner's scalp. Scratch all over the scalp with swift, light movements, keeping your wrists flexible so your nails move loosely from side to side. Make sure that you cover the whole of the head.

Pulsing

For this technique your partner should lie on her back. The weight of the body increases the pressure on the back and neck.

Pulsing eases tired muscles, loosens stiffness in the neck, back, and shoulders, and relaxes the mind and body.

Kneel on the floor at the top of your partner's head. Slide your hands, palms upward, down under the back as far as you can reach. Now make a claw shape with your hands, with fingertips level. Move your hands alternately in small steps, up the back and toward you, so your fingertips apply moving pressure up into the back. When you reach the neck turn your hands so that the neck rests across your index fingers. Moving your hands alternately, lift the neck and pull up and back toward you, smoothly and rhythmically with firm pressure. Repeat for three or four minutes, until you feel the neck relax.

Tapping

This is a light technique that can be used on all areas.

Tapping with one or two fingers can be gentle and soothing, while tapping with all the fingers is very vigorous and stimulating.

Hold your hands so your fingertips are level. Keeping your wrists loose, and with both hands tapping together, bounce your fingertips off the hair with quick, light, smooth movements. Move over the head in regular lines, keeping a regular rhythm.

Hacking

This technique can be used on all areas, but be careful to use only gentle pressure on the top of the head.

Hacking on the back, neck, and shoulders loosens the muscles and encourages deep breathing, while hacking on the head invigorates and stimulates the mind.

Beat with the side of each hand alternately in a light chopping action all over the head, neck, back, and shoulders, keeping a regular rhythm.

Scalp pinching

This technique can be used instead of hair pulling if your partner has very short hair or is balding.

It has the same effect of loosening and releasing tension in the scalp, to relieve tension headaches and to allow the free flow of nutrients to the scalp surface.

Step two
Now place your hand on the top of the head across the midline and pinch the scalp between your thumb and fingers. Hold for three to five seconds. Move back two fingerwidths and repeat. Continue in this way down to the nape of the neck.

Step one
Support the forehead with one hand and place the fingers of your other hand along the hairline at the top of the forehead, just to the side of the midline. Press firmly for three to five seconds. Then with your fingers in the same position, rotate firmly for a count of five. This pressure and rotation loosens the scalp for the pinching. Repeat all over the head in lines, over the top and sides of the head.

Step three
Next, work a line across one side of the head. Stroke over the head for a few moments as you change hands, and then repeat on the other side.

chapter two
Meditation and visualization

Meditation and visualization can help you to relax deeply, allowing your body's own self-healing processes to work. This chapter shows you how to combine these techniques with head massage for effective healing.

Meditation and visualization

Using meditation and visualization with head massage helps you achieve a depth of awareness, stillness, and relaxation that you cannot reach through the physical techniques alone. Together they bring about a completeness in which you and your partner share a unique sense of oneness. This, in turn, greatly amplifies the strength and effectiveness of the treatment.

The dictionary defines meditation as "deep reflection" and visualization as "forming a mental image of something not visible". The difference between the techniques becomes clear if you look at the way both are used in therapy.

During a meditation you focus on an image. This may have color, texture, shape, scent, and some small movement, for example, the candle in the meditation on page 34 in this chapter. Deep concentration and effort are required to achieve a state of relaxed stillness and oneness. In head massage, meditations are used to enhance relaxation, during which the whole of your body is treated to a healing session.

In a visualization your mind travels a journey and your imagination takes you into another reality. From there the visualization seems to take on a life of its own, and your mind and body are carried with it. In the cloud visualization on page 36 your mind is directed to harness the powerful energies of the earth, sky, sun, and water to balance the energies of your body. You can simply allow the healing processes to flow, or you can focus and direct healing to any part of your body, mind, or spirit.

Creative journeying

Visualization has its roots in ancient shamanic traditions, which form a part of many belief systems and ritual practices. True shamans would communicate with animals, plants, rocks, the earth and sky, and other beings, to gain knowledge to help their people. Nowadays hypnotherapy, psychotherapy, and brainstorming sessions all originate from shamanic tradition.

Through visualization you can connect with your subconscious mind, to solve problems, gain different perspectives, or improve your health.

Using the techniques

You can use the meditation and visualization in this chapter as you work through the self-care routine in chapter three, or the complete massage plan in chapter five. These chapters also include other meditations and visualizations: choose whichever appeals to you at the time. For the self-care routine you may find it easier to record the words of the meditation or visualization first and play them as you massage, so your mind can be guided as you work with your hands.

While massaging a partner, talk through the meditation as you work slowly and rhythmically, always maintaining physical and mental contact. Your words and actions should blend seamlessly to create an almost trance-like state in which you are both in tune with the images of the meditation.

First, make sure your surroundings are warm, comfortable, free from distractions, quiet, and peaceful. Lower the lighting, burn incense or oil, play rhythmic, soft music, and allow the rest of the world to go its own way without involving you.

Spend a few moments in silence before starting, to enable you both to connect with the energies of your surroundings. Allow a feeling of ease and comfort to envelop you.

The following breathing exercise prepares you and your partner for the meditation or visualization.

Take a few slow breaths. First, inhale and exhale for a count of three. Then use a count of four. Continue increasing the count by one for each inhalation and exhalation until you reach ten. Then take three more breaths to a count of ten, filling your lungs completely. Now take a long breath and hold it for a count of five before letting it go in a short, sharp burst.

Now forget your breathing; forget everything; just be aware.

Take your awareness to the top of your head, as if you are seeing it as a detached observer. Slowly move it down your body, feeling a wave of warmth flowing down your body as you do so. As the warmth flows through you, you begin to feel more and more relaxed, heavy, and away from the rest of the world.

Now start the meditation or visualization. If your mind drifts to everyday problems, don't fight it. Allow these thoughts to pass through and simply observe them. Slowly they will drift away.

Candle meditation

Imagine a small lighted candle, deep inside your abdomen.

Breathe in, and exhale into the candle flame. The flame grows bigger.

Breathe in and exhale into the flame again. Again it grows. Keep breathing in this way until you can see and feel the candle filling your whole body.

With the next in-breath and exhalation the flame expands beyond your body, extending to about one metre (three feet) outside you.

Now be aware of the warm, golden flame all around you. Don't try to think about it, just feel it.

Observe the flame, noticing that it slowly changes color. You can control this by inhaling and exhaling into the flame.

Stay with each color, breathing gently until you feel at one with it. Feel the healing qualities of each color as it passes over you. Then slowly move to the next.

Breathe in and exhale and the color changes from gold to deep yellow.

When you are ready to move on, take a deep breath and change the color to a soft green. Relax into it.

With the next deep breath and exhalation the color becomes turquoise.

Breathe again and the color deepens to blue.

Now gently change the color to mauve. As you observe the flame this deepens to purple.

Take a breath and the color changes to a crystal clear pink, then slowly deepens to red, and then orange.

With the next breath the orange slowly lightens to yellow and the flame returns to its warm golden glow.

Stay with this golden light until you feel ready to return to everyday consciousness.

When you are ready, allow the flame to grow smaller. With each breath you take, exhale into the flame and see it growing smaller, until it is a tiny light within your abdomen again, containing all the energy and healing power of the colors and light you have seen.

Allow yourself to return slowly to the room and full awareness, feeling refreshed, energized, and wonderfully alive.

Cloud visualization

Imagine you are in the middle of a wood on a warm summer's day. The light is dappled, the shade of the trees is cool and comfortable. Take a while to make this scene as real as you can. See, smell, and feel the different trees, shrubs, flowers, and grasses, the earthiness of the woodland.

Feel your body blending with the character of the surrounding landscape.

Now visualize yourself standing on the bank of a small lake in the heart of the wood. You can see the trees and other plants all around the lake. You can feel the soft muddy ground beneath your feet. You can smell the damp earthiness.

As you look out across the lake you see a mist rising slowly from its surface.

This mist moves toward you and gradually surrounds you. As it swirls around you it feels comfortable, supportive, gentle as the summer breeze. Allow yourself to be supported by the mist. Feel yourself becoming a part of it.

Your body feels lighter and lighter. You are aware that you are growing larger as you become part of the mist. You and the mist are together as one. There is no separation between you and the mist.

You are becoming a loose collection of molecules, drifting higher and higher into the air. You can see the earth far below as you rise higher and higher.

You are spreading out and becoming a soft, light cloud. Feel the tiny atoms of your body that is the cloud. Enjoy this weightlessness and freedom. Feel the energy of the sky, the sun, and the earth below.

Now look down to the earth. You can see the wood and the lake, and a figure standing by the lake. That figure is you.

You are aware that your body is becoming heavier as the cloud condenses to make rain.

You can see tiny rainbows in your body as the raindrops form and the sunlight shines through them.

Gently, you start to fall as rain down on to the wood and the lake.

As you reach the water you can feel yourself forming into a mist floating on the surface.

Lightly, slowly, you float across the water to the figure on the shore.

You feel yourself returning into your body, standing by the shore.

When you are ready, take a few deep breaths and bring yourself back to reality. You will feel energized, refreshed, renewed, and full of light as you come back to the room and become aware of your surroundings.

chapter three

Self-care routine

This self-massage plan shows how to work on your head, back, neck, and shoulders to stimulate the energy throughout your whole body. Use this 20-minute routine daily to invigorate your system.

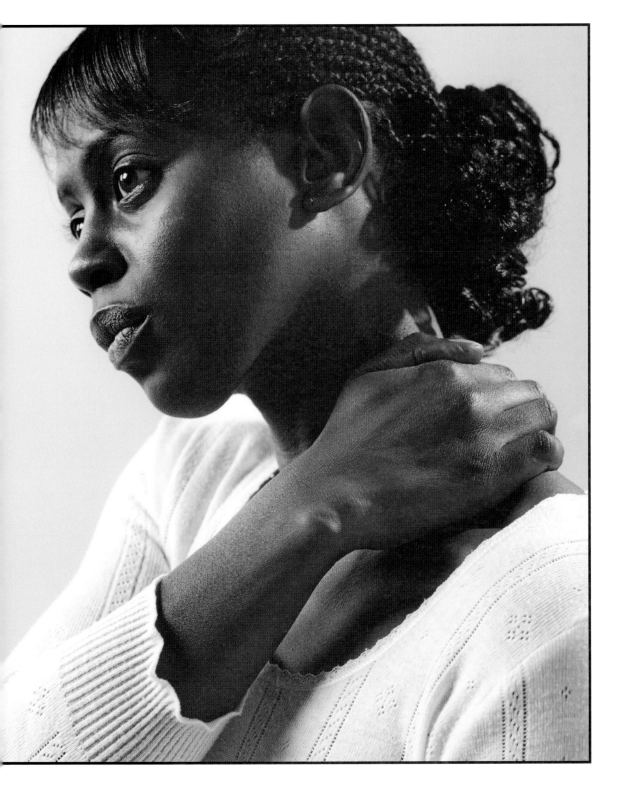

Self-care routine

Before starting the self-care routine, take time to prepare your surroundings: soften the lighting, play soothing music, and burn essential oils (see page 13). Taking time to do this enables you to relax and distance yourself from the rest of the world, thus allowing self-healing to take place.

Now prepare yourself. After centering yourself (see below), follow the golden light meditation on page 41, or use the cleansing visualization on page 14 to create a healing space and reach a place of stillness where you can work effectively.

Once you are familiar with the steps of the routine you may wish to use a simple meditation, such as the water meditation on page 100, as you massage yourself. It may help to record the words of the meditation first so that you don't have to think about it, you can just be.

When you have completed all the steps in the routine, finish with the gold ring visualization on page 56, or the candle meditation on page 34.

Centering yourself

Allow your breathing to become slow and gentle and then spend a few moments observing it, without trying to control it. Consciously become aware of every part of your body. Starting at your head and moving down, look at each part in turn as if you were a detached observer. Notice any tightness and let it go. Take as long as you need for this process.

Caution
Observe the cautions on page 5.

Golden light meditation

Forget time, it no longer exists. The world outside no longer exists.

Imagine that you are floating in the night sky. You are warm and comfortable, weightless and without any particular form. You are aware of your body but it no longer has any constricting boundaries.

Now you can feel a golden light coming toward you from far away in the universe. This is the universal healing energy, coming to renew and regenerate you.

The light enters the top of your head. It fills your head. Feel the power of the light, feel its warmth, color, and vibration.

Allow the light to move down to your neck and shoulders. It relaxes your neck and shoulders. You can feel a warmth moving down your body with the light.

Let the light move down your arms. Feel its strengthening power.

Now the light moves down through your chest and into your abdomen. It fills your body. Warmth and power follow, energizing and healing.

The light moves down your legs and out through the soles of your feet. Feel its surging power.

You are part of a vast golden wheel of light. The light comes down from the universe, through your body, out of your feet, and back up to the universe in a continuous circle.

As the light comes from the universe it brings positive energy into your body. As it returns to the universe it takes with it any negative energy. Stay with this circle for a while. Feel it strengthening and healing.

When you are ready, allow the light to fade gently. Slowly bring yourself back to the room, ready to commence your head massage.

Try to hold on to the stillness of this meditation while you work.

Neck sequence

This massage sequence for the neck will help to keep you supple well into old age. You should only use this technique for self-treatment, as it is easy to overdo it while working on someone else.

Caution
If you have a history of neck problems, you should consult your doctor before using this sequence.

Step two
Starting again at the base of your skull, knead with your fingers down the opposite side of your neck and across your shoulders, along the same line as in Step one. Press as hard as you can. Then change hands and repeat on the other side.

Step one
Clench the fist of one hand and beat with your knuckles on the opposite side of your neck. Work a line down from the base of your skull to the outside edge of your shoulder. Do this as hard as you can bear, two or three times, then change hands and repeat on the other side.

Step four

Again, hold the top right side of your head with your left hand, and place the heel of your right hand on the left side of your chin. This time, push with your right hand and pull with your left, gently tilting your head over to the left, with your ear moving toward your shoulder. Hold for a count of 30, then release slowly and bring your head back upright. Change hands and repeat, this time tilting your head to the right. If you cannot maintain the hold for a count of 30, start with a count of 10 and slowly build up to 30.

Step three

Hold the top right side of your head with your left hand, and place the heel of your right hand on the left side of your chin. Pulling with your left hand and pushing with your right, gently twist your head round to the right as far as you can. Hold this position for a count of 30, then slowly release and bring your head back upright. Change hands and repeat on the other side, this time turning to the left.

Head sequence

Self-massage on the head is invigorating and stimulating. By loosening the muscles of the scalp it helps to prevent tension headaches and also allows blood to flow to the hair roots more easily, improving hair condition. Head massage also affects the pulsing rhythm of the cerebrospinal fluid, allowing it to carry healing messages to other parts of the body.

Caution
Do not use firm pressure on the top of your head if you are elderly, or suffering from epilepsy, bone disease, or clinical depression.

Step one
Start by scratching vigorously all over your head to loosen up your scalp. Then comb your fingers through your hair to remove any knots.

Step two
With your fingers apart, push your hands up into your hair, close to the scalp. Bring your fingers together to grip the hair and pull them out along its length. Hold for three to five seconds, then release. Repeat this pulling, moving your hands slightly each time, until you have covered your whole head.

Step three

Place the pads of the fingers of one hand along the midline on the top of your head, with the little finger on the hairline and the others roughly 1cm (½ in) apart. Rotate your fingers with firm pressure for 3–5 seconds. Move two fingerwidths back along the midline and repeat, continuing until you reach the base of the skull.

Now start again at the hairline and work lines two fingerwidths either side of the midline, using both hands at the same time. Continue in this way, finishing with a line just above the ears. End by rubbing vigorously all over your head.

Head sequence

Step four

Starting at the hairline, in the middle of the forehead, take a small section of hair and pull gently for 3–5 seconds. If your hair is long enough, wrap a small twist around your finger to ensure an even tension. Release, move two fingerwidths back along the midline and repeat the process. Continue in this way until you reach the nape of the neck.

Return to the hairline and, using both hands, work two parallel lines two fingerwidths from the midline. When you reach the neck, run your fingers back up through the hair to ease out your scalp. Then work two more parallel lines back from the hairline. Repeat until you have covered your whole head.

Step five

Comb your fingers through your hair to loosen it. Place the fingertips of one hand along the midline on the top of the head, with your little finger on the hairline and fingers about 1cm (½ in) apart. Press evenly and firmly for 3–5 seconds. Release and repeat, moving four fingerwidths backward each time, until you reach the nape of the neck.

Now start again at the hairline and work back across the head in parallel lines two fingerwidths from the first line, using both hands simultaneously. Try to work smoothly and rhythmically: imagine someone else is doing the work and all you have to do is enjoy it. Continue working parallel lines at two fingerwidth intervals until you reach your ears. Feel the tension draining away.

Step six

Pressure can release tension in a different way when worked from the back of your neck up toward the forehead. This time start at the base of the neck, with the fingers of both hands either side of the spine. Press as hard as you can into your neck and hold for about 5 seconds, then release. Move four fingerwidths up toward the crown and repeat, moving up the neck and on either side of the midline over the top of your head to the hairline.

Now return to the base of the neck and work two parallel lines two fingerwidths from the first. Repeat in this way until you have covered your whole head. Feel the tension lifting from your head.

Caution

Do not apply strong pressure directly on your spine.

Head sequence

Step seven
Tap all over your head with the fingertips of both hands. Your hands should bounce off your hair lightly and rhythmically.

Step eight
Loosely clench your fists and use knuckling to work firmly over your head. Starting at the base of the skull, work from side to side across the back of the head in parallel lines, moving up two fingerwidths each time. Then move to above your ears and do the same on the sides of your head. Finish with a firm knuckling over the top of your head.

Step nine
Scratch your head vigorously all over to complete the work on the scalp.

Ears sequence

There are many acupuncture points in the ears (see page 106). Using pressure and massage on these points balances the energy in your body and internal organs, and also in your mind and spirit. After this technique you may find your hearing is clearer and you feel brighter and more energetic.

Step one
Start at the top of your ears, just where they join your head. Working on both ears simultaneously, pinch the outside ridge as hard as you can, pulling the ears away from your head, and massage slowly between finger and thumb for 3–5 seconds. Release, move one fingerwidth along the ridge, and repeat. Continue all round the outer edge of the ear.

Step two
When you reach your ear lobes, grasp them firmly between index finger and thumb, pulling them down toward your shoulders for 3–5 seconds. Then pull the tops of your ears upward, also for 3–5 seconds.

Step three
Now move into your ears. Use your index finger inside and your thumb behind to pinch and massage all the ridges, nooks, and crannies as firmly as you can. Then work around the outer edge of the ear again, as in Step one.

Eyes sequence

Your eyes contain many muscles and giving them a regular workout can improve your sight. Short sight, long sight, astigmatism, and some focusing problems can all be helped by exercise and massage.

Step one
Start by holding your hands about 20cm (8in) in front of your face, with the palms facing each other 7cm (3in) apart. Be aware of the space between your hands and allow yourself to feel the flow of energy between your palms. Turn your palms to face you, slowly moving them closer to your eyes until you can sense the energy flowing into your eyes. Spend a moment or two with your eyes closed, feeling the strength of the energy flowing into them.

Step two
Still with your eyes closed, tense and relax the muscles within your eyes rhythmically for a count of 20. Then open your eyes and move your hands away from your face, holding one hand at full arm's length, the other about half way. Focus on one hand and then the other, moving quickly between them, for a count of 20.

Step three
Place your palms lightly over your eyes, taking care not to press on the lids. Feel the heat and energy from your palms relaxing your eyes. Tense and relax the muscles for a count of 20.

Step six
Place the tips of the four fingers of each hand beside the outer edge of the eyes, in a vertical line. Rotate them gently as you move your eyes down from the index to the little finger of one hand, and then the other. Repeat this slowly, five times. Finally, relax your eyes by placing your palms over them for 20 seconds, as in Step three.

Step five
Place the tips of the four fingers of each hand in a line under your eyebrows and rotate gently. As you do so, move your eyes along from the tip of one index finger, along the other tips, to the other index finger, and back again. Repeat this slowly five times. Now move your fingers to underneath your eyes, just above the line of the cheekbone. Massage gently with rotations and move your eyes along the line of your fingertips, repeating five times, as before. Rest and relax your eyes by placing your palms over them for 20 seconds, as in Step three.

Step four
Gently massage the bridge of your nose for 2–3 seconds using one finger rotations (see page 19). Look at your finger as you massage, crossing your eyes. Work down the length of the nose and back up again in this way, moving one fingerwidth between positions and following your finger with your eyes. Repeat twice more. Then rest and relax your eyes by placing your palms over them for 20 seconds, as in Step three.

Face sequence

The next steps of the self-care routine work on the face, conditioning the facial muscles and promoting healthy teeth and gums. Facial massage also tones the internal organs and systems via the energy meridians and pressure points on the face (see page 106) and stimulates the lymphatic and endocrine systems (see page 107).

Step one
Start at the base of your throat, with your index, middle, and ring fingers in a horizontal line either side of your larynx. Rotate your fingers firmly for 3–5 seconds, then move up two fingerwidths and repeat. Continue up your throat and under your chin.

Caution
Do not massage your throat if you are pregnant.

Caution
Do not massage the lymphatic areas on the sides of the face, the throat, across the chin, or behind the ears (see page 107), if you have cancer.

Step two
Use your thumbs to make rotations with firm pressure under the jawbone, starting by the base of the ears. Rotate in one position for 3–5 seconds, then move two fingerwidths along the jawbone and repeat, until your thumbs meet in the middle under your chin.

Step three
Next knead firmly along your bottom gums, using the four fingers of each hand. Start in front of your ears, massaging firmly down into the gum for 3–5 seconds and then moving two fingerwidths along the gum line to repeat. Continue until your hands meet on your chin.

Step four
Starting in front of your ears, knead along your top gum as in Step three, this time massaging up into the gum. Your hands should meet just under your nose.

Face sequence

Step six
Use the index, middle, and ring fingers of both hands to rotate firmly in the hollow of your temples for 3–5 seconds.

Step five
Starting in front of the ears again, and using both hands simultaneously, use all four fingers to make light rotations along the cheekbones. Rotate for 3–5 seconds in each position, moving two fingerwidths along each time. Be very gentle under the eyes.

Step seven

Hold the four fingers of each hand so the tips are level and use them to tap firmly all over your face and throat. Work rhythmically with both hands together, keeping your wrists loose so the fingers bounce off your skin.

Caution

Do not massage your throat if you are pregnant.

Step eight

Place the four fingers of each hand on your forehead, in a horizontal line just below the hairline. Feel the muscles in your forehead beneath your fingers, and tense and release these 10 times. The movement is tiny: keep your eyebrows still. Move your fingers two fingerwidths down your face, tensing and releasing the muscles under your fingertips, until you have covered your whole face and throat.

With practice you will become more aware of these muscles and find it easier to tense them.

Gold ring visualization

When you have completed the self-care routine, gently rest your hands side by side on the top of your head with your elbows together in front of your face. Close your eyes and spend a few moments on this visualization, which will help to clear your aura, leaving you energized and refreshed.

You will need to record the words of the visualization first so that you can play them back as you relax.

Illness is believed to appear first in the aura, so using this visualization twice a day, with or without the head massage, will help you maintain good health and wellbeing.

Take a few deep breaths and visualize yourself floating in a clear night sky. Your aura surrounds you as a clear, bright light. Within this light there could appear grey or dark areas.

Move back until you can see the outer limits of your aura. It could be quite compact and close to your body, or it may spread out over a great distance. Make sure you can see it all.

Now see outside your aura a huge spinning gold ring, large enough to surround your aura. Within this ring is a fine gold mesh. As the ring comes toward you the mesh filters through your aura, collecting all the grey or dark patches of negative energy. You can feel yourself becoming lighter as these dark patches are drawn out.

When the gold ring has moved through and out of your aura, close it up with a lid and put another gold ring around it, to seal it. Then see it being taken far away from you into the universe, where the dense negative energy will be transformed into finer positive energy.

Look again at your aura. If there are any dark patches remaining, repeat the visualization until your aura is bright and glowing.

chapter four
Developing the senses

Strengthening your sensory perceptions through the
techniques in this chapter will make you more aware, more
creative, and happier in yourself and your environment.

Developing the senses

The meditations and visualizations in this chapter delve deeply into each area of sensory awareness in turn. Combined with light head massage, they help you develop your senses on a mental, emotional, and physical level. This increased sensory perception will open you to the awareness that everything you need is all around you all of the time – you don't have to cling fearfully to ideas, things, or people. Such an attitude blocks awareness of opportunities just waiting to happen, of people waiting to meet you, so you may miss chances that could enrich your life beyond your expectations.

The only massage technique used is a gentle stroking and touching near the relevant physical parts of your partner's head, while using a meditation or visualization to move her mind through various sensations. If you wish to work through the exercises on your own, record the words of the meditation first so you can concentrate on them completely.

You may want to use these treatments after carrying out the complete massage plan in chapter five, in which case you should move straight into the sense meditation before breaking the energy connection. Alternatively you can work on the senses only, treating one sense per session or combining them for a longer, deeper treatment. If you choose to work this way, omit the last step of each exercise, which brings your partner back to awareness of her surroundings, and continue until you have completed the whole treatment.

For each treatment, position yourself by your partner's head as she lies on the floor. Start by holding the head for a moment as you make the energy connection (see page 88). Talk your partner through the meditation or visualization in a slow, soft voice, allowing pauses between each step to allow her to relax deeply, and following the guidelines given in chapter two.

At the end of the meditation, remember to break the energy connection between you (see page 99).

Touch

Lightly stroke your partner's hair with
alternate hands during this visualization.

Imagine you are walking by a river bank.
Feel the path beneath your feet. Feel the
warmth of the sun, the dappled coolness of
the shady trees.

Sit down on the grass by the river. Feel the
calming rhythms of the earth and the river.

Take off your shoes and put your bare feet
into the cool water. Feel the watery coolness
against your skin.

Run your hands over the grass and the
riverside plants. Feel their different textures
and shapes.

Put your feet on the river bottom. Feel the
plants growing there, the small river-washed
pebbles, the sharpness of the stones.

Sit for a while absorbing all these different
textures, and the feelings and atmosphere
of the river bank.

When you are ready, take your feet out of
the water. Feel the movement of air against
your wet feet. You are back in this room
feeling revitalized and energized.

Taste

Before starting the visualization, spend five minutes on this exercise, which increases the sensitivity of touch and taste within the mouth and can also help improve tongue control for those with speech difficulties.

Ask your partner to breathe through her mouth. Lightly touch her cheek with your finger and ask her to touch her cheek in the same place inside the mouth with her tongue. Hold this position for a few moments while your partner explores all the sensations in the mouth – the feel, the taste, and the breath over her tongue. Move your finger to another position and repeat.

During the visualization, lightly stroke up the sides of the face from the chin to the temples.

Leave fairly long pauses between each step.

Imagine you are walking around a market.

You come to a baker's stall. You can smell the newly baked bread, pastries, and cakes. Sample everything on the stall, and enjoy the variety of tastes and textures.

Next you come to a stall selling herbs and spices. Smell their different aromas – ginger, mint, and cinnamon.

Taste any of the spices you wish.

Move on to the delicatessen stall and sample some exotic foods. Try spicy, sweet, sour, smoked, and pickled tastes.

The next stall sells all kinds of cheese. Try any you like – soft or hard, mild or strong.

Now, walking slowly, retrace your steps through the market. As you pass each stall imagine again all the tastes and textures you have tried.

Take a few deep breaths. As you breathe see if you can still taste all the different foods.

Now slowly come back to this room. Hold on to the richness of all you have tasted.

Smell

Using your index fingers alternately, lightly stroke down your partner's nose from the bridge to the tip during this meditation.

Imagine you are floating in a cloud. It can be any texture, color, or size you wish. If the cloud changes in any way, allow this to happen. Pay particular attention to the scents within the cloud.

First there is a heady smell of roses. It gets stronger and then as the cloud swirls around you, you become aware of other floral scents coming and going. You can choose the scent of any flower – rosemary, lavender, jasmine, sweet pea. Identify each one as it passes.

Other smells swirl around you in the cloud – the wood smoke from a bonfire, freshly cut grass, and damp, earthy smells. Be with each one as it comes and goes.

Now the cloud is full of the smells of foods: spices, coffee, sharp citrus fruits, freshly baked bread. Absorb these scents as they swirl past you.

Feel the changes in the cloud as all the different smells drift by. Enjoy each one. Allow them to come and go.

Pause and take a few deep breaths. Bring your partner's attention back to any scents in the room: aromatic oil, a burning candle, or a vase of flowers.

You are back in this room. Hold on to the variety of all the scents you have smelled.

Hearing

Lightly stroke down the outer ridge of your partner's ears between your index finger and thumb during this meditation.

Imagine you are lying under a shady tree in the middle of a field in summer.

Around you are all the summer sounds of life in this field.

Hear the wind in the leaves of the tree, coming and going in soft gusty breaths.

Hear the songs of the many different kinds of bird in the field.

Hear the insects, the crickets, the bees, the busy life in the grass.

Hear the sound of water far away – a stream splashing over pebbles, or perhaps a river rushing over rocks.

Hear a plane buzzing high above you in the sky.

Hear children playing happily in the field.

Hear the sounds of animals in the fields nearby – cows, sheep, horses.

Pause and take a few deep breaths. Bring your partner's attention back to any sounds in the room, such as a ticking clock.

Hear the cars going past the window. Hear my voice. You are back in this room feeling refreshed and energized.

Sight

Slowly stroke the temples from the corner of the eyes to the hairline during this meditation.

See in front of you a beautiful flower. It is tightly closed, its many layers of petals folded. You are going to open this flower with your breathing.

Breathe in and feel a golden light entering the top of your head.

Breathe out into the flower. The tight bud absorbs this golden light and the petals in the first layer open. They are a bright golden yellow.

Breathe in and now an orange light comes in through the top of your head.

Breathe out and the next layer opens. The petals glow orange.

Breathe in and the light changes to red.

The next layer opens. See and feel the glowing depth of color and energy in the red petals.

Breathe in. Now the light deepens to purple.

The purple layer of petals opens. Feel the healing qualities of this color.

Breathe in. The light changes to blue.

As the layer of blue petals opens, feel your energy lifting.

Breathe in. Now the light is turquoise.

The turquoise layer is now opening. Feel its protection.

Breathe in and a green light appears.

The green, regenerating layer opens.

Breathe in. The green light changes to a bright, golden yellow.

The central yellow petals open. Now the flower is fully formed.

Take a few moments to see and feel this rainbow of color. Feel its healing energy, its strength.

Now allow the flower to close gently within you. Take a few deep breaths, and come back to awareness of the room.

chapter five
Complete massage plan

This massage routine covers the whole head, neck, upper back, and shoulder areas, and is specifically designed to balance energy, tone the muscles, and release tension in the body.

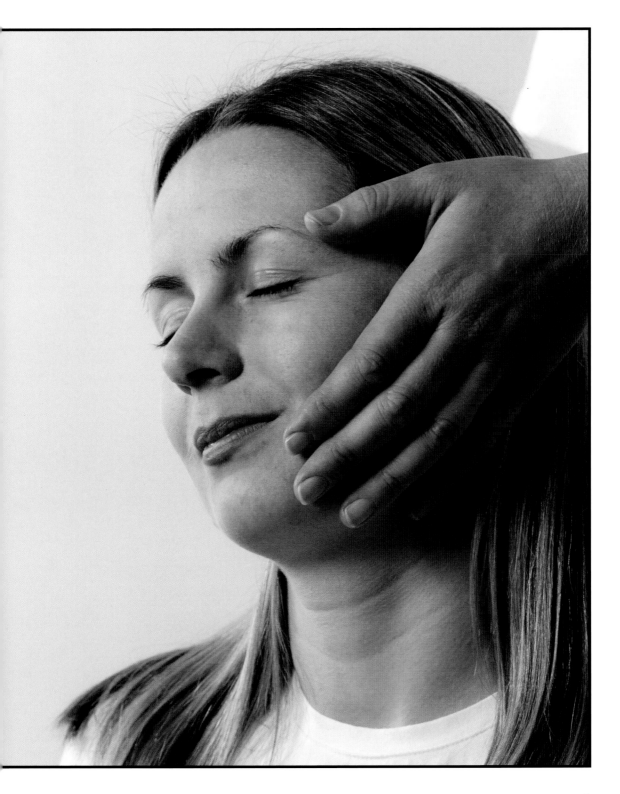

Complete massage plan

The massage plan is given in two versions: one for the sitting position (pages 72–87); the other for lying down (pages 88–99). Each has full step-by-step instructions. Which you choose is up to you. Massage in the sitting position is more invigorating and stimulating for the receiver, while lying down allows the whole body to relax and re-energize.

Both versions of the plan have the same overall benefits for health and wellbeing. The differences in the steps accommodate the different positions of giver and receiver. Both versions tone the muscles and release stress and tension. By stimulating the body's energy meridians and pressure points the massage also balances energy in the internal organs, while stimulation of the lymphatic system boosts immunity, and the endocrine system balances the hormones. Where a step in the massage is particularly effective for certain conditions, this is noted in the description.

Given regularly, preferably once a week, the massage also has a cumulative beneficial effect on your mental state. Relaxation frees up your creativity, so you can deal with day-to-day problems and challenges more easily, and enables the body's own self-healing mechanism to work more effectively.

Both versions of the routine start with centering yourself (described opposite). Using the techniques described in chapter one, they begin with vigorous work on the neck, shoulders, and upper back before moving on to the slower and more meditative head massage. You should start to guide your partner through a meditation or visualization as you move on to the head sequence. Choose from the water meditation or leaf visualization at the end of this chapter, or the candle meditation (page 34) or cloud visualization (page 36) from chapter two.

To work through the complete massage plan will take about 30 to 40 minutes, though it may take longer the first couple of times, while you familiarize yourself with the steps. After massaging your partner you may wish to wait 15 to 20 minutes to ground yourselves before swapping roles.

Once you are confident with the steps of the routine, you can substitute any of the techniques from chapter one, following your intuition.

Caution
Observe the cautions on page 5.

Centering yourself

First prepare your surroundings: soften the lighting, play soothing music, burn essential oils (see page 13), and use the cleansing visualization on page 14 to clear negative energies. Now sit quietly for a few moments and use the golden light meditation on page 41 or the candle meditation on page 34 to center your energy. If you feel at all uncomfortable during the meditation take a break, then a few deep breaths, and start again. When working with a partner it is very important that your energies are harmonious and under control.

Sitting position

Sit your partner in a firm chair with low arms and back and stand squarely behind her.

Making the energy connection

Stand quietly with your thumbs together and palms facing downward, flat on the top of your partner's head. Allow your breathing to synchronize as you make contact with her energies. Close your eyes and visualize a pink healing light coming from the universe down into your head, flowing down your body into your energy center (two fingerwidths below your navel), and then flowing back up your body, along your arms, and through your hands into your partner. Watch this energy moving in a great circle from the heavens, through you both, down into the earth, and then back up to the stars. Try to maintain contact with this energy throughout the massage.

Upper back and shoulders sequence

Tension headaches and eye strain can originate between the shoulder blades, often as a result of poor posture while driving or using a computer, for example. Strong massage releases tension in this area before you start work on the head.

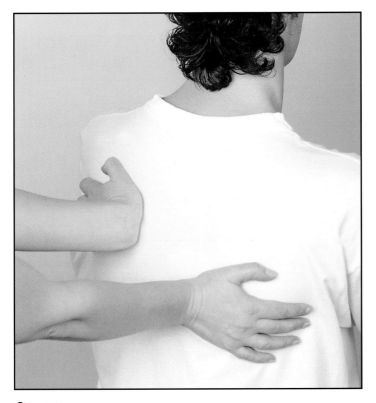

Caution
Do not apply strong pressure directly on the spine.

Step two
Place the pads of your thumbs either side of the spine, level with the lower edge of the shoulder blades. Leaning strongly on to your thumbs, make rotations for 3–5 seconds. Then move your thumbs out two fingerwidths and repeat, working along a horizontal line to the edge of the back. Start the next horizontal line beside the spine, two fingerwidths up from the first, and continue in this way up the back until you reach the neck.

Step one
Position the heels of your hands on either side of your partner's spine, level with the bottom of the shoulder blades. Lean your body weight on to your hands, pushing the muscles outward. Then creep (hand over hand) up the back, parallel to the spine, to the base of the neck, with your hands always in contact with the back. Repeat two or three times to loosen the tension in the upper back.

Upper back and shoulders sequence

Step three
Use strong thumb rotations with downward pressure at two fingerwidth intervals across the tops of the shoulders.

Caution
Do not massage the midpoint of the shoulders of anyone who is pregnant.

Step four
Starting with the heels of your hands either side of the spine and level with the bottom of the shoulder blades, lean and roll in across the heels, at the same time pushing the muscles outward. Work across the back in lines, up to the base of the neck, as in Step two.

Step five
Clench your hands into fists and use strong pressure and a rolling action to knuckle up the upper back, pushing the muscles outward from the spine. You can work hand over hand all over one side and then the other, or else use both hands simultaneously to work in lines out from the spine over the whole upper back (see Step two).

Shoulders and upper arms sequence

Following the steps below helps to release locked or stiff muscles in the shoulder area, thus enabling the neck to move more freely. It also encourages deeper breathing.

Step one

Place the backs of your forearms at the base of your partner's neck, on either side of the head. Your hands should face upward, fists loosely clenched. Lean down strongly for a count of five.

Now rock your body back, move your arms four fingerwidths away from the neck and lean down again. Repeat this action across the shoulders until you reach the tops of the arms.

Caution

Do not massage the midpoint of the shoulders of anyone who is pregnant.

Step two

From your position in Step one, rotate your forearms inward so your fists face each other. Keeping a strong pressure, slide your forearms down the outside of your partner's arms to the elbows. Repeat twice more, then rub all over the arms, back, and shoulders.

Neck sequence

Tension in the neck can aggravate headaches, eye strain, and focusing problems. Releasing this tension can relax the whole body.

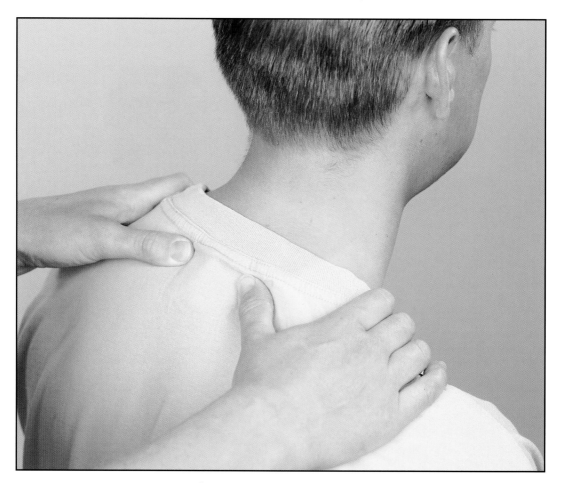

Step one
Place your hands on the shoulders with your thumbs either side of the spine at the base of the neck. Leaning your weight on to your thumbs, use thumb rotations to work up the neck on both sides of the spine, two fingerwidths from the midline, until you reach the base of the skull. Keep the pressure firm and even throughout. Repeat twice more.

Head sequence

Massage on the head releases tension in the scalp and improves blood circulation to the hair. Using these techniques slowly and rhythmically enables your partner to reach a very deep state of relaxation.

Caution
Do not use firm pressure on the top of the head on the very young, the elderly, or anyone suffering from epilepsy, bone disease, or clinical depression.

Step two
Stroke lightly all over your partner's hair with the palms of your hands. Then comb through the hair loosely with your fingers apart and relaxed, separating the hair but not touching the scalp. These soothing movements are used throughout the treatment to keep a smooth, flowing rhythm as you change from one technique to another.

Step one
With your hands on either side of your partner's head, hold the head lightly until your breathing synchronizes. This steadying action after the strong work on the shoulders and neck prepares you both for the more relaxing part of the massage routine. As you hold the position, re-establish your connection with the universal healing energy. Visualize a clear, bright light from far above you, passing through your body into your partner's body, and down into the earth.

Now start to talk your partner through the water meditation on page 100, or the leaf visualization on page 101.

Head sequence

Step three

Support the forehead with one hand, and use two fingers of the other hand to make rotations from the hairline back along the midline at one fingerwidth intervals. Work over the top of the head and down to the base of the skull. Here press upward with both fingers for a count of three. Return to the hairline and work a parallel line two fingerwidths from the first line. Finish by pressing upward at the base of the skull for a count of three. Continue until you have covered one side of the head. Stroke the hair for a few seconds, then change hands and repeat on the other side of the head.

Step four

Starting at the base of the skull, stroke and comb up through the hair toward the hairline, working over the scalp in the opposite direction to the rotations in Step three.

Step five

Hold your fingers with your nails in line and lightly scratch all over the head, keeping your wrists loose. This technique is invigorating and very good for skin conditions such as dandruff and psoriasis.
Stroke or comb through the hair for a few moments.

Caution

Do not work on broken skin, or sore areas of the scalp.

Step six

Support the head with one hand, and use one finger of the other hand to apply pressure for 3–5 seconds at one fingerwidth intervals along the midline. Start at the hairline and work back over the head to the nape of the neck, or work in the opposite direction if you prefer. Then work over one side of the head in the same way, in parallel lines two fingerwidths apart. Stroke the hair lightly and change hands to work on the other side of the head. This technique is excellent for heavy headaches, tension, and eye strain. Stroke or comb through the hair, from the nape of the neck to the hairline.

Head sequence

Step seven
Using both hands at the same time and keeping to a regular rhythm, tap all over the head. Keep your wrists loose and bounce off the scalp. This can be done lightly or vigorously, as your partner prefers.
Comb your fingers gently through the hair to remove any knots.

Step eight
Starting with your hands on either side of the neck, slide them up into the hair, fingers apart, keeping close to the scalp. When you have gathered a handful of hair, close your fingers firmly and pull away from the head. Allow the hair to move through your fingers under tension, creating a strong, even pull. Repeat all over the head, always pulling the hair at right angles away from the scalp.
Stroke or comb through the hair, from the nape of the neck to the hairline.

Step nine
Support the forehead with one hand.
Make a fist with the other and knuckle
up the neck and back of the head in a
vertical line. Then work a parallel line,
two fingerwidths from the first, over
the side of the head. Stroke all over
the hair, then change hands and
repeat on the other side.

Step ten
Support the forehead with one hand.
With the heel of the other hand, knead
with strong pressure up the back of
the neck and head to the crown. Then
start at the neck again, this time
kneading up over the side of the head.
Stroke the hair as you change hands
and knead up the neck and over the
other side of the head. Then knead the
top, from crown to forehead.
Rub all over the head briskly, then
gently comb or stroke the hair.

Throat sequence

Massage on the throat tones the neck muscles and also boosts the immune system by stimulating the lymphatic areas either side of the throat (see page 107).

Caution

Do not massage the throat of anyone who is pregnant or has cancer.

Step one
Rest your hands gently at the base of the throat for a moment or two. Reconnect with your partner's energies by visualizing the universal healing energy coming into your energy center, as on page 72. Now use your fingers to stroke up the throat and round under the ears, using alternate hands with brisk, light movements for about 30 seconds.

Step two
Working with both hands together, make two finger rotations gently up the throat, either side of the midline. Repeat on parallel lines two fingerwidths from the first. Then start under the chin and use four fingers to rotate firmly along the jawbone to the ears, moving two fingerwidths between rotations.

Face sequence

These techniques condition the facial muscles and promote healthy teeth and gums. Through the energy meridians, pressure points, and the lymphatic and endocrine areas on the face (see pages 105–107), face massage also tones and stimulates the internal organs, boosts the immune system, and balances the hormones. For these techniques use both hands on either side of the face simultaneously.

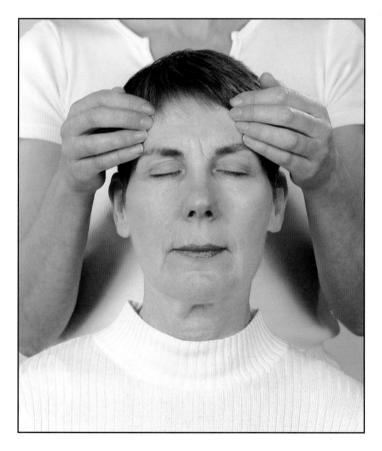

Caution
Do not massage the lymphatic areas on the sides of the face, the throat, across the chin, or behind the ears (see page 107), on anyone who has cancer.

Step one
With light, brisk finger movements, stroke up the sides of your partner's face from the jaw to the temples. Now work across the forehead with four finger rotations. Start in the middle with your fingertips in a vertical line and work outward with both hands, moving two fingerwidths between positions and rotating for 3–5 seconds on each point.

Face sequence

Step two

Starting in the middle of the chin, work along the jawbone with one finger rotations, one fingerwidth apart. Repeat in parallel lines at two fingerwidth intervals up over the cheeks, finishing on the cheekbones. Now return to the middle of the chin and use firm two finger pressure under the chin for 3–5 seconds. Repeat along the jawbone, moving two fingerwidths each time.

Step three

Use one or two fingers to knead along the lower gums, moving outward and back from the middle. Knead for 3–5 seconds in each position before moving two fingerwidths to the next. Then repeat along the upper gums. This technique stimulates blood flow to the gums and encourages healthy teeth.

Step four
Hook all four fingers gently under the
cheekbones and hold this position for
3–5 seconds. Then do the same under
the eyebrows.

Step five
Now apply firm pressure into the skull
with all four fingers on the forehead,
just above the eyebrows.
These techniques help sinus conditions
and can lift heavy headaches.

Ears sequence

Massage on the ears balances energy in the body, mind, spirit, and the internal organs through stimulation of the acupuncture points illustrated on page 106. Use both hands for these techniques, to work on both ears simultaneously.

Step one
Starting at the top of the ears where they meet the head, and pinching between index finger and thumb, rotate all around the outer edge. When you reach the lobes, pinch them firmly and pull them down toward the shoulders for 3–5 seconds.

Step two
Rub the ears briskly then cup your hands over them for 3–5 seconds. They will probably be quite hot and your partner may hear a ringing or buzzing sound, which should fade after a few moments.

Breaking the energy connection

Finish the treatment by holding your partner's head firmly but gently with your hands on either side. Visualize the clear white light of healing energy flowing down from the universe into your head, through you and your partner, down into the earth, and back up again to the stars, in a huge circle.

Now see this flow of white light being cut above your head. Remove your hands from your partner, holding them 2–3cm (1–1½in) above her head. See the light flowing down through your body, through your partner, out through the bottom of your feet, and into the earth. Step back and stamp your feet, breathing deeply to ground yourself. This breaks the energy connection between you.

Lying down

Thoroughly pad the floor with a duvet, sleeping bag, or folded blankets. Your partner should lie on her back for the massage. Make sure you have some padding to sit on too. Kneel or sit on the floor above and close to your partner's head, so that you can comfortably reach down the back of her neck and under her shoulders.

These back, neck, and shoulder techniques can be replaced with the techniques from the sitting position section of this chapter if you prefer.

Making the energy connection

Sit quietly with your hands resting either side of your partner's head. Allow your breathing to synchronize as you make contact with her energies. Close your eyes and visualize a pink healing light coming from the universe down into your head, flowing down your body into your energy center (two fingerwidths below your navel), and then flowing back up your body, along your arms, and through your hands into your partner. Watch this energy moving in a great circle from the heavens, through you both, down into the earth, and then back up to the stars. Try to maintain contact with this energy throughout the massage.

Upper back and shoulders sequence

Tension headaches and eye strain can originate between the shoulder blades, often as a result of poor posture while driving or using a computer, for example. Strong massage releases tension in this area before you start work on the head.

Step two
Use the heels of your hands to knead across the tops of the shoulders, from the neck outward to the top of the arms, and back again.

Caution
Do not massage the midpoint of the shoulders of anyone who is pregnant.

Step one
Holding your hands flat, with the palms facing upward, reach down under your partner's back as far as you can. Make a claw shape with your hands, then start next to the spine and move both hands out toward the sides in a horizontal line.
Your partner's body weight increases the pressure in this powerful technique. If you can, repeat twice more in parallel lines two fingerwidths apart.

Neck sequence

Tension in the neck can aggravate headaches, eye strain, and focusing problems. Releasing this tension can relax the whole body.

Caution

If you have a history of neck problems you should consult your doctor before using this sequence.

Step one
Hold your hands together under the base of the neck, so that it rests on your index fingers. Keeping your hands together, pull strongly upward and toward the nape of the neck. Repeat twice more.

Step two
With your hands in the same position as Step one, change to a hand over hand action, still pulling in the same direction. This rolling movement will rock the head gently from side to side. Continue for a count of 20, to loosen the neck muscles.

Hold the back of your partner's neck until your breathing synchronizes. As you hold the position, re-establish your connection with the universal healing energy by visualizing a clear, bright healing light from far above you in the universe passing through your body, into your partner's body, and down into the earth.

Now start to talk your partner through the water meditation on page 100, or the leaf visualization on page 101.

Head sequence

Massage on the head releases tension in the scalp, and improves blood circulation to the hair. Using these techniques slowly and rhythmically enables your partner to reach a very deep state of relaxation.

Caution
Do not use firm pressure on the top of the head on the very young, the elderly, or anyone suffering from epilepsy, bone disease, or clinical depression.

Step one
Gently stroke upward all over your partner's hair. This soothing movement is used throughout the treatment to keep a smooth, flowing rhythm as you change from one technique to another.

Step two
Turn your partner's head to one side and support the neck with one hand, letting the head rest on your forearm. Work a line up the middle of the back of the neck and head to the crown, using two finger rotations with one finger either side of the midline. Rotate for 3–5 seconds at each point, moving two fingerwidths between points. Work a second line two fingerwidths from the first, up the neck, and over the side of the head.
Now turn the head to the other side and repeat the two finger rotations up the midline and then over the side of the head.

Head sequence

Step three

Turn your partner's head to the front
and slide your hands under the back
of the head as far as you can reach.
Work up the sides of the head to the
temples, using four finger rotations at
two fingerwidth intervals.

Step four

Now support the side of the head
and use the four fingers of one hand
to make rotations over the top of the
head in one big sweep from the crown
to the forehead. Gently stroke or comb
through the hair for a few moments.

Step five
Slide your hands under the back of the head as far as you can reach. Use the four fingers of one hand to press firmly for 3–5 seconds. Work up the sides of the head in this way, moving two fingerwidths between positions and finishing at the temples.

Step six
Starting at the temples, use firm thumb pressure to work a line in across the middle of the forehead, holding each position for 3–5 seconds and moving one fingerwidth to the next. Finish where your thumbs meet in the middle.

Head sequence

Step seven
With your thumbs overlapping, use thumb pressure to work a line from the middle of the forehead down to the crown. Hold the pressure for 3–5 seconds on each point and move back two fingerwidths between positions. Then use one thumb on each side of the head to work two lines, two fingerwidths from, and parallel to, the first line; then on two lines from the "corners" of the forehead. Gently stroke or comb through the hair for a few moments.

Step eight
Starting as far toward the back of the head as you can reach, scratch lightly all over the scalp, keeping your wrists loose so that the movement is light, free, and flowing.

Step nine
Use the four fingers of both hands to tap all over the head, starting as far back as you can reach and moving up over the sides. Try to work in regular lines, and keep your wrists loose so your fingertips bounce off the head. Work either lightly or vigorously, as your partner prefers. Then support the head and tap over the top, from crown to forehead and back again, using the backs of the fingers. Comb through the hair with your fingers to loosen any knots or tangles.

Step twelve
Knead simultaneously up both sides of the head to the temples, so the pressure from each hand balances the other. Use an open hand, and knead with pressure from the heel of the palm to the base of the fingers. Then support the head with one hand and knead over the top with the other, as for knuckling in Step eleven.

Step eleven
Starting as far down the back of the head as you can reach, knuckle up and over both sides of the head at the same time, finishing at the temples. Then support the head with one hand while you knuckle over the top with the other, rolling across the knuckles from side to side and moving forward from the crown to the forehead.

Step ten
Turn your hands so that the palms face outward, spread your fingers, and push them down through the hair at the sides of the head. When you have gathered a handful of hair, close your fingers to grip it and then pull slowly away from the head, letting the hair move through your fingers under tension. Repeat this step in a smooth, flowing manner all over the head, always pulling the hair at right angles to the scalp.

Face sequence

These techniques condition the facial muscles and promote healthy teeth and gums. Through the energy meridians, pressure points, and the lymphatic, and endocrine areas on the face (see pages 105–107), face massage also tones and stimulates the internal organs, boosts the immune system, and balances the hormones. For these techniques use both hands on either side of the face simultaneously.

Caution
Do not massage the lymphatic areas on the sides of the face, the throat, across the chin, or behind the ears (see page 107), on anyone who has cancer.

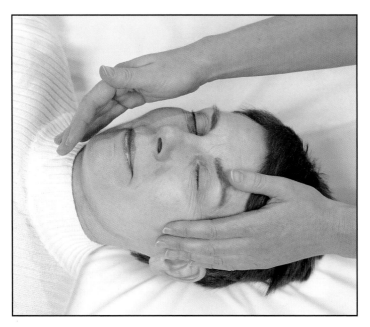

Step one
Using alternate hands, stroke up the throat and sides of the face toward the temples in a continuous motion. Do this for 10 seconds, then stroke very lightly with the fingertips from the chin up to the cheekbones, and then on the forehead, avoiding the eyes.

Step two
Use the four fingers of both hands to tap lightly up the throat and over the face toward the temples.

Step four
Use your thumbs to knead along the lower gum, starting at the back of the jaw and meeting under the middle of the lower lip. Knead each position for 3–5 seconds, before moving one fingerwidth to the next. Then repeat along the upper gums. This technique stimulates blood flow to the gums, and encourages healthy gums and teeth. Stroke the face lightly with your fingertips. Work from the middle out to the ears, on the forehead, beside the nose, and on the chin.

Step three
Hook four fingers under each eyebrow and press gently with the fingertips for 3–5 seconds. Release, then hook under the cheekbones in the same way and press again. Then do the same under the jawbone, with your index fingers together under the chin and your other fingers spread out along the jaw.

Step five
Start with the four fingers of both hands in a horizontal line across the base of the throat. Rotate gently for 3–5 seconds, then move up two fingerwidths and repeat, until you reach the chin.
Now start at the jawbone and continue using four finger rotations up the cheeks to the temples. Then start again above the eyebrows and use four finger rotations to work up the forehead to the hairline. Use light pressure without pulling the skin. Stroke gently with your fingertips up both sides of the face to finish.

Ears sequence

Massage on the ears balances energy in the body, mind, spirit, and the internal organs through stimulation of the acupuncture points illustrated on page 106. Use both hands for these techniques, to work on both ears simultaneously.

Step one
Starting at the top of the ears where they meet the head, and pinching between index finger and thumb, rotate all around the outer edge. When you reach the lobes, pinch them firmly and pull them down toward the shoulders for 3–5 seconds.

Step two
Rub the ears briskly, then cup your hands over them for 3–5 seconds. They will probably be quite hot and your partner may hear a ringing or buzzing sound, which should fade after a few moments.

Breaking the energy connection

Finish the treatment by holding your partner's head firmly but gently with your hands on either side. Visualize the clear white light of healing energy flowing down from the universe into your head, through you and your partner, down into the earth, and back up again to the stars, in a huge circle.

Now see this flow of white light being cut above your head. Remove your hands from your partner, holding them 2–3cm (1–1½in) above her head. See the light flowing down through your body, through your partner, out through the bottom of your feet, and into the earth. Move back away from your partner. Take some deep breaths and shake your hands vigorously. This breaks the energy connection between you.

Water meditation

This meditation allows your partner to reach a state of deep relaxation while you work at a slow, meditative pace. Speak in a slow, soft, gentle but firm voice.

Vary the pauses between sentences so that you reach the long pause as you begin to massage the ears.

Be aware of your breathing. Feel your breath gently moving into your body and back out again.

Feel your breath slowly filling your whole body each time you inhale.

Feel the tension in your muscles leaving your body each time you exhale.

Breathe in. Feel your body becoming softer and softer.

Breathe out. Feel your body slowly dissolving.

You are becoming lighter and more fluid with each breath.

See yourself glowing with a soft rainbow colored light.

Your body is becoming lighter, you are floating. Your body is spreading out, you are becoming like the surface of a lake.

As the lake is blown by the warm breeze, the sun creates tiny rainbows within the ripples.

Stay with this feeling of liquid, light, and color. Let these feelings develop. Allow any changes in your body and mind to happen.

Long pause…

As you come to the end of the massage, start speaking again.

Now feel your body becoming more dense. You are becoming yourself once more.

Feel your body re-forming, bringing with it the power and energy of the water, colors, and the sun.

Now you should be at the end of the treatment, holding your partner's head as you break the energy connection between you.

Take a few deep breaths and come back to awareness.

Leaf visualization

This is an excellent grounding visualization which can help to stabilize an over energetic mind and body. While you work, imagine you are also within this visualization and simply describe everything that happens to you. This script is only a guide.

Vary the pauses between sentences so that you reach the long pause as you begin to massage the ears.

Take a few breaths to center yourself.

As you observe the air moving in and out of your body, feel yourself spreading out, becoming very light, very flexible, boneless.

Feel yourself drifting in a cool breeze. You are very loose. You are being wafted up and down, from side to side. You are so light you are being carried by the gentlest of air currents.

Feel yourself moving like a leaf on the topmost branch of a tall tree.

Look down and see the ground far below. Enjoy floating in the air with just the faintest connection between you, the tree, and the earth.

Now put your awareness into that connection. The stem joining you to the tree brings you life, strength, and power.

Feel the power of all living things moving through you.

Feel the power of the tree drawing you toward it.

Feel the hard, woody texture of the tree as you become part of it.

You are becoming stronger as you move into the branch.

You are moving along the branch and into the trunk of the tree, absorbing the strength and vitality of the tree and the earth beneath.

Feel every sensation – the flow of energy, health, power. You are being reconstructed as you feel the power of life growing within you.

Long pause…

Now you should be at the end of the treatment, holding your partner's head as you break the energy connection between you.

Now slide down the tree, and out on to the ground. Be aware of your breathing. Feel yourself coming back to reality. Start to be aware of your surroundings as you return, feeling strengthened and regenerated.

chapter six
Treating common ailments

The step-by-step treatment plans in this chapter show you how
to use the power of head massage to promote healing for
25 common ailments and conditions.

Treating common ailments

The plans in this chapter give a comprehensive general treatment for 25 ailments and conditions, working on the channels and areas illustrated on the following pages. Refer back to these illustrations as you follow the treatment plans.

The exact position of channels, areas, and points varies from person to person, therefore the illustrations should be used as a guide.

Channels

The free and balanced flow of energy in mind, body, and spirit maintains good health. This energy flows along channels that are related to the body's organs or functions. Massage on these channels frees blocked energy, balancing energy flow in the related organ system.

Most of the channels occur in pairs, symmetrically on either side of the body. Not all of them extend as far as the head, but some, such as the lung channel, have an extension channel in the neck and head area which can be treated in the same way as the channel itself.

In the treatment plans in this chapter you will notice that some massage points seemingly unrelated to the problem are used to stimulate the healing process. For example, respiratory problems respond to massage on the bladder channel. This is because the respiratory system is part of a vast network that deals with elimination. This includes the digestive system, blood circulation, bowels, bladder, tears, sweat, nail and hair growth, skin and cellular replacement at all levels, and even emotions. If there is a problem in the respiratory system, stimulating other systems concerned with elimination, such as the bladder, takes the pressure off the weakened respiratory system, allowing it to recover.

Key

■ large intestine channel

■ stomach channel

■ spleen extension channel

□ gall bladder channel

■ lung extension channel

□ bladder channel

Still points

Along the base of the skull are still points which can be used to slow the heart rate, deepen breathing, lower blood pressure, assist with lymph drainage, and deeply relax the body. Since lymph can transport some forms of cancer cells around the body, these areas should not be massaged on anyone who has cancer.

Pressure areas on the face

Some areas on the face relate to specific organs, for example the pancreas points, which are located either side of the middle of the chin. Massage on these areas tones and balances the related organ system.

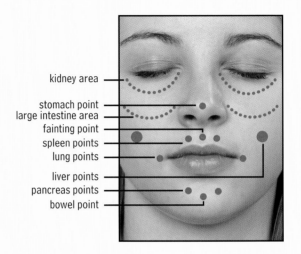

kidney area

stomach point
large intestine area
fainting point
spleen points
lung points

liver points
pancreas points
bowel point

Pressure points in the ears

Acupuncturists use over 200 points in the ears to treat all parts of the body and mind. Treating these with pressure, as in finger and thumb massage, is known as acupressure. Since fingers and thumbs are quite blunt instruments, massaging in the ears allows you to stimulate several points at once.

Massaging all over the ears benefits the whole being, regulating the digestive system, improving immunity, clearing the breathing, lowering blood pressure, and detoxifying.

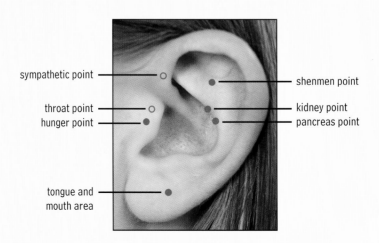

sympathetic point

throat point
hunger point

tongue and
mouth area

shenmen point

kidney point
pancreas point

The endocrine system

The body responds to stressful situations by releasing hormones such as adrenaline and cortisol. Massage on the endocrine areas (see right) stimulates the pineal, pituitary, and thyroid glands to balance hormone levels. This helps to counteract the negative effects of stress, which is a major component of many ailments and conditions.

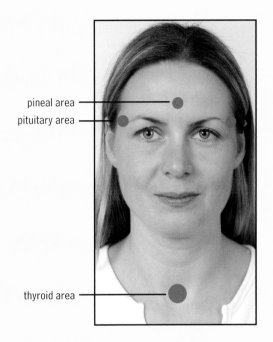

pineal area

pituitary area

thyroid area

The lymphatic system

Lymph (a clear fluid) travels through the body via the lymphatic system, clearing toxins. It is a major component of the immune system, so massaging the lymphatic areas on the sides of the face, the throat, across the chin, and behind the ears, strengthens immunity. Since lymph can transport some forms of cancer cells around the body, these areas should not be massaged on anyone who has cancer.

Balancing the body's energies

General head, neck, and shoulder massage is a wonderful way to relax and de-stress the body, mind, and spirit. Since stress imbalance aggravates almost every ill, relaxing and balancing stress levels promotes general wellbeing. In addition to stress overload, many ailments are also greatly aggravated by the build-up of toxins within the body, energy and hormone imbalances, and reduced immunity.

Relaxing mind and body enables the self-healing mechanisms to work at maximum efficiency. Detoxing frees more energy for cellular repair and regeneration. Your skin becomes clearer, you feel more alive, your mind and body feel more in tune and energized.

The treatment plans in this chapter all include relaxation and detox techniques relevant to the particular ailment being treated, in addition to other beneficial massage steps and a visualization that specifically promotes healing of the condition. You can follow these plans to treat yourself, though the treatment will be more effective if a partner gives you the massage, thus allowing you to concentrate fully on the visualization. All the treatments are safe to use on both adults and children, though you should only ever use a light touch on the very young or elderly, and observe the cautions given on page 5. Always start by working through the complete massage plan in chapter five, stopping just before you break the energy connection with your partner, and then continuing with the appropriate treatment plan.

Treating ailments

The techniques for treating ailments and conditions work on the channels and areas illustrated on pages 105 to 107. However, many different points and channels can be massaged to achieve the same result, and some may work better than others, depending on the individual. Also, people have their own preferences – some do not like having their faces massaged, others may have extra sensitivity in the neck or throat. Once you feel confident with the steps suggested, if you feel that your partner would benefit from work on a particular area, or that a particular massage technique would be more effective, go with it. Work

Caution
The treatments in this chapter are safe and effective but are not intended to replace the care of a qualified medical practitioner. Do not make any changes to your existing treatment or medication without consulting your doctor. Observe the cautions on page 5.

intuitively, with love and care and a desire for the wellbeing of others, and you will give more healing than if you try to stick to a regimented format.

During the treatment it is important to keep the energy moving. Otherwise, although you may damp down the symptoms, a build-up of energy may cause a blockage, which could lead to problems later. Visualize a white, violet, or pink light around the problem while you work. At the end of the session, as you break the energy connection between you, see this light flowing down your partner's body, out of the soles of the feet, and away into the universe.

The healing crisis

When you use head massage treatments you may find you seem to get worse before you get better. This is because the therapy is getting to the root of the problem, not merely suppressing the symptoms.

Delving into a problem can disturb a lot of deeply buried discomfort and can also reveal emotional pain. Experiencing a release in body or mind, pain, or dreaming and reliving past events are fairly common reactions to treatment.

Many people give up at this point, preferring to leave the discomfort as quickly as possible. Stick with it if you can, and use the pain to clear out deep-seated problems. You can then rise beyond your old self into a new, positive, creative, energetic, and exciting you.

Detox

Toxins in our everyday environment can include pollutants in the air, pesticides on our food, and chemicals in cleaning products. Natural substances can also be toxins: too much fat or sugar in a rich meal, or too much alcohol. Stress reduces the body's natural ability to cope with such toxins, and signs of toxic overload may include skin or hair problems and other minor ailments.

These treatments stimulate the elimination systems to rid the body of toxins and balance the hormonal system. Many of the treatments in this chapter include this detox routine, since reducing toxins allows the body's healing mechanism to cope with the underlying cause of the illness.

▲ **Step one**
Use finger rotations along the stomach and large intestine channels (see page 105). Rotate firmly and slowly on each position for 10–30 seconds, moving back two fingerwidths each time. Massage in the same way along the bladder channel (see page 105).

▲ **Step two**
The midpoint of the chin is the bowel point (see page 106). Massage here for 10–30 seconds with firm thumb rotations. Then use finger rotations on the end of the nose (the stomach point, see page 106) for 10–30 seconds.

Visualization

Visualize a white light coming down through the top of your head. Slowly it fills your head, neck, shoulders, arms, and hands. Now the light moves into your body, filling all the organs, then down into your legs and out through the soles of your feet. Feel this light flowing in a continuous movement through your body, picking up grey areas of negative energy, and moving them out through the soles of your feet, down into the earth.

▲ **Step three**

Put your index finger in the ear, with the edge of the nail aligned with the ear hole. Slide it up until it meets the inner ridge and then rock the finger back: the pad of the finger will now be on the kidney and pancreas points (see page 106). Massage with pressure for 10–30 seconds to stimulate the kidneys and regulate salt and sugar levels in the blood.

▲ **Step four**

Tap gently with one finger around the eye sockets below the eye, from the nose around to the outer corner. This area relates to the kidneys, bowels, and large intestine. Then use firm finger rotations, pressure, and tapping over the middle of the forehead, the temples, and the base of the throat, to balance the endocrine system.

Headaches

The most common cause of headache is tension, which often originates in the shoulders, leading to tight muscles in the neck and scalp. Sinus problems may cause head pain across the forehead and cheeks. Bilious headaches may result from overeating, or too much rich food or drink. Regular head massage relaxes the shoulders, neck, and head.

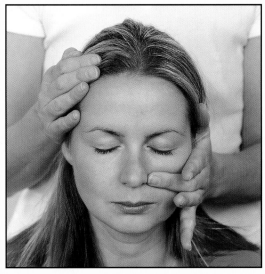

▲ Treatment one

For tension headaches, use strong scalp, neck, and shoulder massage. Starting on the shoulders, work up the neck and all over the scalp, using thumb rotations, heel of hand kneading, pressure, hacking, hair pulling, and tapping. This loosens tight muscles and releases pain.

Hair pulling can also be very effective for this type of headache. As you work over the scalp you may find painful hot spots. Grasp the hair over the affected area and hold it under tension for 10–20 seconds, then release. This relaxes the muscles of the scalp and can make a headache vanish in seconds.

▲ Treatment two

For sinus headaches, massage either side of the nostrils with the pad of your middle finger, resting it under the cheekbones. Apply firm pressure along the length of the finger for 5–10 seconds, then use rotations at one fingerwidth intervals. Follow this with finger pressure along the cheekbones, holding for 5–10 seconds before moving along one fingerwidth to the next point. You can also use finger pressure on the middle of the bridge of the nose. This is particularly useful if the cheekbones are tender.

Caution

Do not use these techniques on anyone who has had surgery to drain the sinuses.

▲ Treatment three

To lift a fuzzy headache and to relieve any head pain, massage the sympathetic point on the ear (see page 106). This is near the top of the ear, close to where it joins the head. Slide your finger under the outer ridge and press on the inner end of the horizontal ridge. Your partner should breathe deeply as you massage this area as you will find her mind clears very quickly.

Treatment four

To clear toxins, use the detox massage treatment plan on pages 110–111.

Visualization

Imagine a gold ring spinning and encircling your body around your energy center (two fingerwidths below your navel). Allow it to rise up your body, and up from the top of your head, moving the pain with it, up and out of your body.

Migraine

Migraine headaches result from tension and physical stress in the membrane around the brain and the muscles of the scalp. Causes of such tension may include stress, eyestrain, hormone imbalances, infection, neck and back problems, allergy, excesses of food or alcohol, and depression.

Do not use head massage during an attack, as it can intensify the discomfort. Instead, use these treatments once or twice a week as a preventive measure, to reduce the frequency of attacks.

▲ Treatment one
To balance the endocrine system, massage the middle of the forehead (pineal gland), the temples (pituitary), and base of the throat (thyroid) with two finger rotations for 10–30 seconds on each. If your partner finds rotations too strong, use stroking instead.

Treatment two
To release tension in the scalp and membrane around the brain, use stroking, rotations, and light pressure all over the head, working in regular lines. Then work horizontal lines on the neck, shoulders, and upper back with kneading and strong thumb rotations. Finish by tapping lightly over all these areas.

Treatment three
To clear toxins, use the detox massage treatment plan on pages 110–111.

Visualization

Imagine lying under a lime tree in early spring. The day is warm and you can see the sky through the pale green and yellow leaves. The blues, yellows, and greens flow through you, draining away all tension and pain.

Neuralgia

This localized nerve pain commonly affects the cheek and gum areas, but may also occur in the throat and ears, or on other areas of the body, for example with shingles. Other possible causes are stress, emotional upset, vitamin deficiencies, and excess alcohol.

Massage affected areas daily to reduce pain. If you suffer recurrent attacks, use these techniques twice a week until the incidence is reduced, then weekly as a preventive measure.

▲ Treatment one
To relieve pain, use rotations and pressure to massage firmly in lines across the forehead from the middle out to the temples. Then work along the cheekbones to the bridge of the nose using tapping or rotations. Massage each point for 10–30 seconds before moving to the next. Stroke lightly from the middle of the forehead to the temples, then back along the cheekbones to the nose. Treat other affected areas similarly.

Treatment two
To release tension in the facial muscles, massage the back of the neck with strong thumb rotations, working out from either side of the spine in horizontal lines.

Treatment three
To clear toxins, use the detox massage treatment plan on pages 110–111.

Visualization

Feel your head surrounded by a bright yellow cloud. Ice-blue shards move through the cloud. When one comes close, feel its coolness drawing the pain away. As the pain drifts away, the ice melts and the blue and yellow mingle. Stay with this calming, healing, pale green colour.

Sleep disturbance

Problems with sleeping have many causes, including emotional disturbance, digestive problems, allergies, and overstimulation, for example from watching television last thing before bed.

Working through the complete massage plan twice a week calms and reduces stress, helping the mind to organize information. Use once a week when symptoms improve.

Treatment one
Strong thumb rotations up the back of the neck will help to relax the mind. To release tension across the shoulders, firmly knead the upper back and shoulders with the heels of the hands, then follow with thumb rotations and pressure. In both these areas work in lines out from the middle, massaging for 10–30 seconds on each point.

▲ Treatment two
Calm the mind by massaging the shenmen point in the ear (see page 106). This is on the edge of the dimple just below the outer ridge at the top of the ear, at this dimple's furthest point from the head. Pinch firmly with your thumb behind the ear and finger inside and massage with rotations for 10–30 seconds.

▲ Treatment three
To slow down mind and body and coax your partner into relaxed sleep, use light rotations slowly and repetitively on the endocrine areas: the middle of the forehead, the temples, and base of the throat (see page 107).

Visualization

Feel yourself floating high in the sky as the sun is setting. The sky is filled with yellows, oranges, purples, and pinks. Feel the warm air all around. As the sky darkens and the blue deepens, feel yourself falling into a calm, restful sleep.

Caution
Do not massage these areas on anyone who has cancer.

▲ Treatment four
Massage with upward stroking, four finger rotations, and pressure in lines over the lymphatic areas on the throat, under the jaw, the sides of the face, and the back of the neck (see page 107).

Treatment five
To clear toxins, use the detox massage treatment plan on pages 110–111.

Hyperactivity

This condition can be aggravated by allergies, emotional upset, low immunity, toxin build-up in the body, and brain damage.

Daily treatment can promote calm and encourage mental relaxation. Use only light pressure if treating children.

Follow the treatment plan for sleep disturbance, but use firm pressure on the endocrine areas, to balance the hormones rather than promote sleep.

Visualization

Imagine floating on the surface of a mountain lake. Feel the deep blue water cooling and calming you. Allow your body to dissolve over the surface of the lake. Stay with the calm, relaxing, floating feelings.

Depression and anxiety

Common causes include emotional problems, childbirth, reactions to childhood experiences, and responses to pain or stress that get out of control. Anxiety has similar symptoms to depression, along with an element of fearfulness.

Regular head massage with meditation or visualization calms the mind and promotes a positive self-image.

▲ Step one

Relax the scalp using slow, gentle stroking, combing, and light hair pulling all over the head, over and over again. This will take your partner to a deep level of relaxation where her mind and body can let go. Here she needs support rather than stimulation: understanding love and a safe environment in which to release.

Caution

Do not use firm pressure on the top of the head on the very young, the elderly, or anyone suffering from epilepsy, bone disease, or clinical depression.

▲ Step two

Once your partner is deeply relaxed, hold the head with one hand on the back of the neck and the other on the forehead and guide her through the visualization on the opposite page.

▲ Step 3

Without coming back to the room from the visualization (see right), move on to massaging the shenmen point in the ear (see page 106) for about five minutes as you talk your partner through the candle meditation on page 34. It is the most important point for calming the mind. Pinch firmly with your thumb behind the ear and finger inside, and massage with light rotations.

Visualization

Feel around you a warm, golden glow. Smell the scent of lavender. As you become more aware of the warmth, light, and scents around you, the glow becomes infused with a soft violet light. Allow this light to move slowly into your being. Feel the light reaching through to your heart. Stay with this light. Feel its healing and protection.

Mental exhaustion

Tension can lead to a continuous tensing of the muscles in the neck, upper back, shoulders, and head. This in turn can cause headaches, backache, tight scalp (preventing circulation of blood and nutrients to the hair), tiredness, mental fatigue, and mind and body burnout. The immune system becomes suppressed, leaving the body open to attack from physical, mental, and emotional problems.

Weekly head massage relieves stress, encourages sleep and eating patterns to stabilize, and gives you more energy to cope with stressful situations.

Meditation

Imagine floating in a warm, comforting pink and gold cloud.

▲ Treatment one

To balance and strengthen the immune system, massage each of the lymphatic areas (see page 107) for 10–30 seconds. First work up the front of the throat with four finger rotations in horizontal lines. Then use four fingers under the jaw, spreading the fingers to cover the length of the jawbone. Now use four finger rotations behind the ears and around to the base of the skull, followed by light finger kneading and four finger pressure.

Caution

Do not massage these areas on anyone who has cancer.

▲ Treatment two

To stimulate and balance the endocrine system, massage the temples and middle of the forehead with two finger rotations for 10 seconds followed by firm pressure for 10 seconds. Then massage the thyroid area at the base of the throat (see page 107) with two finger rotations for 10 seconds.

▲ Treatment three

As an instant energy booster, pinch the kidney and pancreas points on the ear (see page 106) between thumb and index fingernails and massage for 10–30 seconds. To find these points, put your index finger in the ear, with the edge of the finger nail aligned with the ear hole. Slide it up until it meets the inner ridge and then rock the finger back: the pad of the finger will now be on the kidney and pancreas points. Massage on these points may be painful, but it gives a powerful energy lift.

Chronic fatigue syndrome

Symptoms of this debilitating condition, also known as myalgic encephalomyelitis (ME), include lack of energy, depression, muscular pains, headaches, nausea, and memory loss. Among the suspected causes are viral infection, immune imbalance, psychological or neurological problems, and overuse of antibiotics.

Regular head massage improves feelings of wellbeing, reduces stress, helps to counteract feelings of fatigue and depression, and boosts the immune system.

As someone suffering from this condition may not want to be bothered with massage, you may want to begin with gentle stroking and combing combined with a light meditation, and gradually work up to a full head massage, introducing new techniques each time.

Heart and circulatory conditions

These are aggravated by high blood pressure, excess weight, stress, emotional problems, and imbalances in energy, immunity, and the hormones. In particular, high blood pressure adversely affects the heart muscles, and conditions such as angina and palpitations, as well as accelerating the narrowing of the arteries.

Regular head massage, following the complete plan in chapter five, helps to reduce blood pressure and lower stress levels. It deeply relaxes the muscles, reducing blood vessel constriction and improving the circulation.

Visualization

See a soft pink light all around your heart. As you relax, feel this light moving through your arteries, veins, and capillaries, healing and strengthening them. Hold this image for as long as you can before allowing it to be absorbed slowly by the rest of your body.

▲ Treatment one

If your partner is sitting down, support the forehead firmly with one hand. With the thumb and fingers of your other hand either side of the spine, rotate strongly up the neck toward the head. When you reach the top of the neck, push with slowly increasing pressure in an upward direction in the hollow just under the base of the skull. At the same time resist the push with your supporting hand. Hold for 20 seconds. You may find your partner's breathing deepens.

Repeat the whole movement twice more, widening your grip on the neck by one fingerwidth each time. This will cover three still points on either side of the spine (see page 105). Finish with a gently rotating massage over the back of the neck.

Treatment two

If your partner is lying down, work rotations with four fingers either side of the neck, with the little fingers next to the spine and the others in a line parallel to the shoulders. This enables the whole neck to be treated in one go. When you reach the base of the skull, hook your fingers under the bony ridge and pull toward you with slowly increasing pressure. A gentle shaking movement at this point encourages the whole body to release tension.

Caution

Do not massage the lymphatic areas on the sides of the face, the throat, across the chin, or behind the ears (see page 107), on anyone who has cancer.

Excess weight

Underlying causes of excess weight can include stress, emotional problems, eating disorders, low self-image, and negative childhood experiences.

Used regularly, this treatment improves self-image, reduces stress, and combats cravings. The visualization can be used during the massage, or whenever food cravings occur.

▲ Treatment one
To reduce cravings rotate firmly with a fingertip or nail on the hunger point, in the hollow immediately in front of the ear (see page 106). This is a quick and easy treatment which can be used whenever cravings occur.
Also, to calm the mind, massage the shenmen point in the ear (see page 106). Pinch firmly with your thumb behind the ear and finger inside and massage with light rotations.

▲ Treatment two
Massaging the lung points at the corners of the mouth (see page 106) with finger rotations or pressure, will help to move negative emotional patterns and improve self-image.

Treatment three
To clear toxins, use the detox massage treatment plan on pages 110–111.

Visualization

See before you a delicious, fattening food. Feel yourself becoming heavy just by looking at it. Now see the food shrinking. As it becomes smaller and smaller you feel lighter and lighter. See it now as small as a pea in your hand. You feel light and free. You no longer see this food as interesting. Let it go.

Digestive problems

Irritable bowel syndrome, stress-related diarrhea, indigestion, constipation, flatulence, and peptic ulcers can all be aggravated by stress, depression, anxiety, negative emotions, and hormone imbalance.

Regular head massage relaxes mind and body, reduces stress, and restores hormone balance, therefore allowing the digestive system to relax, and harmonizing its function.

▲ Step one
Massage with two finger rotations, pressure, tapping, and stroking at two fingerwidth intervals along the gall bladder channel (see page 105).

▲ Step two
Then use finger pressure for 10–30 seconds on the pressure areas for the liver (in the middle of the cheek, pictured above), the kidney points, and the pancreas points (see page 106).

▲ Step three
Press with the length of your fingers along the cheekbones for 10–30 seconds to treat the large intestine area. Then use finger pressure for 10–30 seconds on the bowel point (see page 106).

Step four
To clear toxins, use the detox massage treatment plan on pages 110–111.

Visualization

Imagine you are inside a cool, deep turquoise block of ice. Feel the coolness calming your body through to the center. As your body relaxes, feel the ice melting. Feel bubbles releasing from the ice as it melts. (At this point, if you feel you need to release trapped wind, do so.) As the ice melts it changes to a glowing golden light all around and through you, healing, calming, and regenerating you.

PMS and menstrual problems

Almost 200 symptoms are related to PMS and menstruation. Among the most common are headaches and migraine, low energy, digestive and skin problems, cravings, disturbed sleep, poor concentration, depression, and mood swings.

Regular head massage can rebalance hormones, reduce stress and toxin levels, and boost energy.

During menstruation, concentrate on the orange and the blue in the meditation below, feeling the healing power of the colors moving through you.

Treatment

To balance hormone levels, work on the endocrine areas – the base of the throat, temples, and middle of the forehead – with stroking, rotations, pressure, and tapping. Spend more time within the red of the rainbow meditation (below). This will help to boost your energy and calm mood swings, while supporting and healing your whole being.

Meditation

Imagine you are floating around in a rainbow, feeling the vibration of each color as you move through it. From yellow into orange lifts your mood. From orange to red energizes you and shifts tiredness. The strong healing color purple strengthens you. From the purple change to blue, calming and soothing. Float through to turquoise. You may feel a release within you. Now to green – a healing, calming, and renewing color. The green lightens and becomes a golden yellow. You feel refreshed and regenerated.

Pregnancy

Common pregnancy problems such as nausea, high blood pressure, heartburn, tiredness, and back pain can be eased by head massage. Treatments help balance hormones, boost immune and digestive systems, and calm body and mind.

In the first three months of pregnancy use only stroking, combing, and other light techniques. Later you can use stronger techniques on the back, but the massage should still be lighter than usual.

Use the rainbow meditation on the previous page, spending extra time within the green to help calm the mind.

Caution

In pregnancy do not massage on:
- *the spleen points (see page 105)*
- *the spleen extension channel (see page 105)*
- *the gall bladder area (see page 105)*
- *the midpoint of the shoulders (a point on the gall bladder channel)*

Baby massage

Gentle massage is soothing and relaxing for parent and child, encouraging a strong bond between them. A traditional part of childcare in many cultures, massage stimulates healthy development and has been shown to promote growth in premature babies.

Treatment

Lie your baby across your lap, face down, and stroke with your fingers down the back of the head and along the back. Then, with your baby sitting against your chest, rest your fingers on the baby's shoulders and use your thumbs to stroke gently down over the side of the head. Stroke lightly over the top of the head with your fingers. Keep your movements light and flowing.

Skin conditions

Your skin, more than anything else, reflects your inner being. Conditions such as eczema, dermatitis, psoriasis, acne, and non-infectious skin rashes can all be improved by reducing stress, detoxing the body, and boosting the immune and endocrine systems.

Regular head massage, particularly with strong work across the back, shoulders, neck, and scalp, deeply relaxes the body, enabling its self-healing systems to rejuvenate and repair the skin.

Caution

Do not massage on broken skin or infectious skin rashes.
On sore areas stroke lightly, or hold your hands 1–2in (2–3cm) over the area, focusing healing energy on to it.

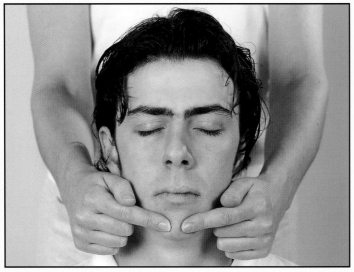

Meditation

Imagine yourself surrounded by an aura – an energy cloud of pale yellows, blues, greens, and pinks.

▲ Treatment one
Massaging the pancreas points on either side of the middle of the chin (see page 106) for 10–30 seconds helps to balance blood sugar levels.

Treatment two
To boost immunity, enabling the skin to defend itself more easily, massage the throat, sides of the face, in front of and behind the ears, and down the back of the neck with stroking, four finger rotations, pressure, and tapping.

Caution
Do not massage these areas on anyone who has cancer.

Treatment three
To balance the hormones and calm the mind, use one or two finger pressure, rotations, stroking, and tapping on the endocrine areas – the temples, middle of the forehead, and base of the throat (see page 107).

Treatment four
To clear toxins, use the detox massage treatment plan on pages 110–111.

Mouth and throat problems

Inhaled pollutants, allergens, bacteria, and viruses all enter the body through the nose, mouth, and throat. If you have a tendency to suffer from mouth and throat problems, such as cold sores, oral thrush, toothache, tonsillitis, and laryngitis, this can be aggravated by stress and low immunity.

Use these treatments regularly after a full head massage as a preventive measure, and also to speed recovery from sore throats and other mouth problems.

▲ Treatment one

To stimulate cellular repair in the throat area, massage on the throat point (see page 106). With your finger inside the ear and thumb outside, use pressure and rotations on the underside of the tragus (the gristly flap in front of the ear) for 10–30 seconds.

Treatment two

Calm the mind by massaging the shenmen point in the ear (see page 106). This is on the edge of the dimple just below the outer ridge at the top of the ear, at this dimple's furthest point from the head. Pinch firmly with your thumb behind the ear and finger inside and massage for 10–30 seconds.

▲ Treatment three

To relieve muscular tension and pain in the mouth and throat, pinch the mouth area on the earlobe (see page 106) and rub it between finger and thumb for 10–30 seconds.

Treatment four

The body is less able to cope with pollutants and other toxins if it is already suffering from toxin overload. To clear toxins, use the detox massage treatment plan on pages 110–111.

Visualization

Visualize cool blue water all around you. Feel yourself floating within a sea of healing energy. As you relax, the water becomes a deeper and deeper blue. Stay with the cooling, healing energy of this water.

Respiratory problems

There are many causes of respiratory problems, including viral and bacterial infections, allergies, smoking, irritants such as dust, emotional upset, and hormone changes.

Regular head massage can help to reduce the intensity of attacks in conditions such as emphysema, bronchitis, asthma, catarrh, hay fever, and sinus problems. By relaxing mind and body it gives the self-healing systems a chance to work, and also boosts energy, strengthens the immune system to fight infection, and rebalances the hormones.

Caution
Do not massage these areas on anyone who has cancer.

▲ Treatment one
To strengthen the lungs, massage the lung pressure points on the outer corners of the mouth (see page 106). Use your index finger to make rotations with firm pressure for about 30 seconds.

▲ Treatment two
An extension to the lung channel runs up the throat, two fingerwidths either side of the windpipe (see page 105). Use rotations with light pressure to massage up both sides of the windpipe simultaneously, treating each point for 30 seconds before moving two fingerwidths up to the next.

Treatment three
To boost the immune system, massage the sides of the face, under the jaw, behind the ears, in the hollow at the back of the neck, up the throat, and over the chin. Use stroking, gentle four finger rotations, and light pressure, all pressing in an upward direction over this whole area.

▲ Treatment four
To help relieve the congestion, stiffness, and feverishness that accompanies a cold, massage up the back of the neck on either side of the spine. Use rotations and pressure, working outward in horizontal lines from the middle. If your partner is lying down, place your hands under her neck and use pulsing and stretching.

Treatment five
Strongly massaging up the neck and over the upper back will help the lungs to cope with an asthma attack. Use thumb rotations either side of the spine up the neck, and heel of hand kneading and thumb rotations to work up the spine in horizontal lines, always working outward from the middle.

Treatment six
The lungs are part of the elimination system (see page 104) and so detoxing will help to clear any toxin overload they have to cope with. Use the detox massage treatment plan on pages 110–111.

Visualization

Visualize holding a bright orange marigold. Feel the joyous power in the color. Feel it brightening and clearing your head and chest. Slowly it turns to a clear yellow, calming, and strengthening. Feel all its power and energy moving through you.

Muscular problems

The body contains two types of muscles: voluntary, which control the movements of the limbs for example, and involuntary, which control the movements of the internal organs. Stress puts the whole muscular system under tension, and prolonged stress is the root of many muscular problems.

Head massage relaxes the muscles. When it is combined with visualization, which convinces your involuntary muscles that you are in a safe environment, your body can let go and move into a state of repair and rejuvenation.

Treatment one
Some hormonal imbalances may cause muscle weakness. Massage the endocrine areas at the base of the throat, temples, and the middle of the forehead (see page 107), using stroking, rotations, pressure, and tapping for 30 seconds in each area.

▶ Treatment two
Strong massage of the back, neck, shoulders, and scalp following the routine in chapters three or five, encourages the body to relax and release tension, and improves the circulation. A strong, vigorous treatment is particularly effective for muscle pains and strains anywhere in the body, for stress-related backache, and for problems such as repetitive strain injury (RSI). You may have to start gently and build up to a strong massage if your partner finds the treatment painful. Use the visualization on the opposite page.

Rheumatism

This is usually taken to mean any disorder that results in pain in the muscles and bones. It can be caused by inflammation of the muscles and is exacerbated by stress, lack of sleep, and emotional upset.

To reduce stress and emotional upset, give regular full head massage following the routines in chapters three or five.

Treatments for sleep problems are on pages 116 and 117.

Arthritis

Arthritic pain arises from inflammation of the tissues in the joints. This inflammation has various causes, including wear and tear on the joint, stress and tension in the muscles, poor circulation, reduced immunity, and a build-up of toxins within the joints and muscles.

Regular head massage reduces stress and tension, rids the muscles of toxins, and improves circulation.

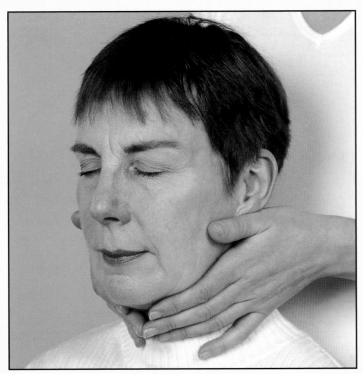

Visualization

Imagine you are sitting in a rose garden in early summer. Close your eyes and be aware of the scents around you. Now gaze at the wonderful colors all around: reds, yellows, oranges, pinks and mauves. Feel their healing energy within your body and mind.

▲ Treatment one
To boost the immune system, stroke lightly up the throat, sides of the face, over the chin, and in front of and behind the ears.

Treatment two
To clear toxins, use the detox massage treatment plan on pages 110–111.

Caution
Do not massage these areas on anyone who has cancer.

Hair and scalp problems

Alopecia or baldness has many causes, including stress, poor circulation, pregnancy, chemotherapy, iron deficiency, and toxin overload. Regular head massage reduces stress, releases toxins, relaxes the scalp, and improves circulation, stimulating the supply of nutrients to the hair roots. Treatment can also prevent dandruff, which can occur when the oils in the scalp are unbalanced and a yeast infection builds up.

The massage should be vigorous and stimulating. There is no visualization to accompany this treatment, since stronger techniques make concentration difficult.

▲ Step one
To loosen the muscles and release constriction around the hair roots, use strong massage on the upper back, shoulders, and neck. Use thumb rotations with firm pressure either side of the spine, working up from the level of the shoulder blade at two fingerwidth intervals.

Then push the muscles out and away from the spine with heel of hand kneading, working up the back in horizontal lines, two fingerwidths apart. Use your body weight to apply pressure to move the muscles so that they become loose, flexible, and relaxed. Hack all over the upper back to give a stimulating finish.

▲ Step two
Now work on the shoulders. Start with the backs of your forearms close to either side of your partner's neck and lean your weight down strongly. Move to a position four fingerwidths toward the arms and repeat.

Now start close to the neck again and work all over the shoulders with thumb rotations and then pressure. Finish with hacking over the shoulders.

Caution
Do not massage the midpoint of the shoulders of anyone who is pregnant.

▲ Step three
Use the strong, vigorous techniques such as rotations, pressure, kneading, hair pulling, scratching, and hacking to work all over the scalp. For people with little hair, or a very short haircut, use the techniques on page 29.
On the neck, work strongly up either side of the spine, with thumb rotations, pressure, and kneading.

Caution
Do not apply strong pressure directly on the spine.

▲ Step four

To strengthen the hair, stimulate circulation, and loosen the scalp, grasp two handfuls of hair, very close to the scalp on the top of the head, and move the scalp backward and forward about 2cm (1in). Repeat on the sides and back of the head. Some people have very tight scalps so you may have to work up to full strength gradually.

Additional treatments

For a very effective anti-dandruff treatment, crush an aspirin and mix it with your regular shampoo. Use once a week.

If your hair is dry or damaged, oils can help bring back the shine and condition. Work a little coconut oil through the hair at the end of the massage and leave it on for 24 hours before shampooing out. Macassar oil is also effective, and is found in some shampoos.

Tinnitus

Sufferers usually hear a ringing, buzzing, roaring, hissing, or whistling noise in one or both ears, and sometimes there is also hearing loss. Causes include injury to the head or ear, infection, toxin build-up in the body, high blood pressure, or heart problems. Stress and muscular tension in the back, neck, and shoulders can make tinnitus worse.

Regular head massage helps to reduce blood pressure, which can lead to a reduction in noises in the ear.

▲ Treatment one
To loosen muscular tension and improve the circulation, use strong massage on the back, shoulders, and neck. Use thumb rotations, leaning in with your body weight to increase the pressure, up either side of the spine on the back and neck, and across the shoulders. Work up the back in horizontal lines using heel of hand kneading from the middle outward. Lean in and push the muscle away from the spine.

Caution
Do not massage the midpoint of the shoulders of anyone who is pregnant. Do not apply strong pressure directly on the spine.

▲ Treatment two
To calm the mind and reduce stress, use hair pulling, pressure, tapping, hacking, and rotations all over the top of the head.

Caution
Do not use firm pressure on the top of the head on the very young, the elderly, or anyone suffering from epilepsy, bone disease, or clinical depression.

Treatment three
To clear toxins, use the detox massage treatment plan on pages 110–111.

Visualization
See a gold light surrounding your head. Feel this light penetrating into the ear. The light drains the noise from the ear, out and away.

Eye strain

Stress and tension in the neck, shoulders, and back of the head affect the muscles in the eyes, so they work less effectively. Therefore before starting to treat the eye area you should thoroughly loosen these areas, following the routine in chapter three. Then use the techniques for the eyes on pages 50 to 51. These tone and condition the muscles in your eyes and, practised daily, can improve your eyesight.

▲ **Treatment one**

To strengthen the eye muscles, massage round your eye sockets, starting at the bridge of the nose and following a figure of eight. Use very light one finger rotations, working on each point for 2–3 seconds before moving on. Follow your finger with your eyes and complete five circuits before resting your palms over your eyes and relaxing for 5–10 minutes.

Treatment two

Your eyes will become tired if you focus at one distance for some time, for example when reading or looking at a computer screen. To relax them, focus on something in the distance – a view through a window for example – and then move your focus back to something closer, such as the glass in the window. Alternate between the two up to 20 times, holding the focus for one breath in each position.

Epilepsy

Fits or seizures result from a sudden burst of abnormal electrical activity in the brain. Regular head massage, using only a light touch and a lot of stroking and combing in an upward direction, soothes and helps to reduce stress, while meditation promotes calm and relaxation.

Caution

Do not use firm pressure on the top of the head on the very young, the elderly, or anyone suffering from epilepsy, bone disease, or clinical depression.

Visualization

Imagine you are lying in long, green grass. The day is warm and you feel comfortable and relaxed. Allow the green of the grass to permeate your body, bringing a loose, calm feeling to your mind and body.

▲ Treatment one
Calm the mind by massaging the shenmen point in the ear (see page 106). Pinch firmly with your thumb behind the ear and finger inside and massage using rotations for 10–30 seconds.

Treatment two
To clear toxins, use the detox massage treatment plan on pages 110–111.

Fainting

For cases of fainting, keep the person lying down to encourage blood flow to the brain and massage the point one fingerwidth above the middle of the upper lip using strong rotations. Remove any false teeth, or the treatment can be painful. The person should soon regain consciousness.

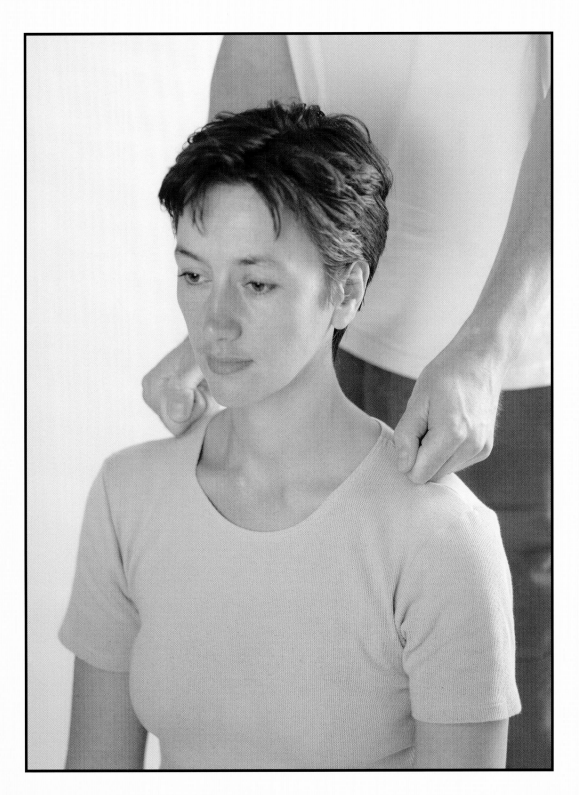

Author's acknowledgements

I would like to express my grateful thanks to all my relatives, friends, students, and teachers who have helped me, in many ways, to complete this book. I would like to thank all at Gaia Books for their hard work and support. I would like to thank fate for its gift of broken bones which, at just the right moment, freed my time for writing.

Publishers' acknowledgements

The publishers would like to thank: Helena Petre and Charlie Ryrie for editorial assistance; Kitty Crossley, and Owen and Jenny Dixon for design assistance; Jackie Beazer, Eilean Bentley, Anne Brabyn, Vicky Eggleton, John Ganly, Sharon Hamilton, Mike Harding, Geoff Hitchings, Adrian Lee, Hazel Morbey, Wilk Morbey, Tom Morbey, Charlotte Morgan and Katherine Pate for modelling; and Lynn Bresler for the index.

Photographic credits

All photography by Steve Teague except: pages 34 and 67 Delilah Dyson; pages 61 and 65 David Woodfall, Woodfall Wild Images; page 63 all Telegraph Colour Library; page 64 Marie O'Hara.

Eilean Bentley

Bibliography

Angelo, Jack
Your Healing Power
1998, Piatkus

Bach, Edward
Heal Thyself
1996, Beekman

Brennan, Barbara Ann,
Hands of Light
1993, Bantam Doubleday
Dell

Devananda, Swami Vishnu
Meditation and Mantras
1978, OM Lotus Publishing

Horan, Paula
Empowerment Through Reiki
1990, Lotus Light
Publications

Horan, Paula
Abundance Through Reiki
1995, Lotus Light
Publications

Honervogt, Tanmaya
The Power of Reiki
1998, Owl Books

Jarmey, Chris; Mojay, Gabriel
Shiatsu, The Complete Guide
1992, Thorsons

Jarmey, Chris; Tindall, John
*Acupressure for Common
Ailments*
1991, Fireside

Kando, Juliette
Natural Facelift
1991, Thorsons

Lam, Master Kam Chuen
The Way of Energy
1991, Fireside

Lundberg, Paul
The Book of Shiatsu
1991, Fireside

Shen, Peijian
*Step-by-Step Massage for
Pain Relief*
1996, Random House

For information about a CD
of meditations or a video to
accompany this book, please
contact:

Gaia Media
20 High Street
Stroud
Gloucestershire
GL5 1AZ
UK

00 44 (0)1453 752985
or:
eileanbentley@lineone.net

Index

Explosive Lifting for Sports

Harvey Newton

Human Kinetics

Library of Congress Cataloging-in-Publication Data

Newton, Harvey.
   Explosive lifting for sports / Harvey Newton.
       p. cm.
   Includes index.
   ISBN 0-7360-4172-9
       1. Weight training. I. Title.

   GV546 .N49 2002
   613.7'13--dc21

2001051637

ISBN: 0-7360-4172-9

Acquisitions Editor: Ed McNeely; **Developmental Editor:** Cassandra Mitchell; **Assistant Editor:** Dan Brachtesende; **Copyeditor:** Patsy Fortney; **Proofreader:** Erin Cler; **Indexer:** Sharon Duffy; **Permission Manager:** Toni Harte; **Graphic Designer:** Robert Reuther; **Graphic Artist:** Tara Welsch; **Photo Managers:** Tom Roberts and Carl Johnson; **Cover Designer:** Keith Blomberg; **Photographer (cover):** Tom Roberts; **Photographer (interior):** Tom Roberts, unless otherwise noted; © Bruce Klemens pp. 45-48, 52-53, 57-58, 62-64, 80-82, 98-99; figure 7.3 © International Weightlifting Federation; **Art Manager:** Carl Johnson; **Illustrator:** Tom Roberts; **Printer:** United Graphics

Human Kinetics books are available at special discounts for bulk purchase. Special editions or book excerpts can also be created to specification. For details, contact the Special Sales Manager at Human Kinetics.

Printed in the United States of America   10   9   8   7   6   5   4   3

Human Kinetics
Web site: www.HumanKinetics.com

United States: Human Kinetics, P.O. Box 5076, Champaign, IL 61825-5076
800-747-4457
e-mail: humank@hkusa.com

Canada: Human Kinetics, 475 Devonshire Road, Unit 100, Windsor, ON N8Y 2L5
800-465-7301 (in Canada only)
e-mail: orders@hkcanada.com

Europe: Human Kinetics, 107 Bradford Road, Stanningley
Leeds LS28 6AT, United Kingdom
+44 (0) 113 255 5665
e-mail: hk@hkeurope.com

Australia: Human Kinetics, 57A Price Avenue, Lower Mitcham, South Australia 5062
08 8277 1555
e-mail: liaw@hkaustralia.com

New Zealand: Human Kinetics, Division of Sports Distributors NZ Ltd.
P.O. Box 300 226 Albany, North Shore City, Auckland
0064 9 448 1207
e-mail: blairc@hknewz.com

Contents

Acknowledgments

Since I first mounted the competition platform at age 15, weightlifting has provided me a great number of rewards and opportunities. First as an athlete, later as a coach, and finally as an administrator, weightlifting and strength training have always been a large part of my life. Along the way I've made great friends and worked with outstanding colleagues. All of them deserve strong thanks.

From local clubs and clinics to the US Olympic Training Center and beyond, athletes from many different sports and all levels of accomplishment have added to the challenge and enjoyment of teaching explosive-style weightlifting. A heartfelt thank-you for the many opportunities you have provided.

Explosive Lifting for Sports provides a great opportunity to share ideas with readers I'd never meet otherwise. Thanks to Michael Mahoney, who years ago encouraged me to write a book on weightlifting. Thanks to Rainer Martens and Human Kinetics for the opportunity to finally do so. A special thanks to my acquisitions editor Ed McNeely, developmental editor Cassandra Mitchell, and assistant editor Dan Brachtesende, who have patiently and professionally supported me throughout this experience. Thanks to all the great HK staff who have contributed to this book.

Tracy Fober deserves special praise as a fresh source of information and support throughout this project.

This book would not have been possible without the great competition photographs of Bruce Klemens. "Köszönöm" to Ms. Aniko Nemeth-Mora, of the International Weightlifting Federation, for her photographic support as well. HK's Tom Roberts worked hard to get the exercise technique pictures just right. Special thanks go to York Barbell Company and the St. Louis Weightlifting Club for the gracious use of their facilities.

I truly appreciate the coaches who contributed their insights into how they utilize explosive lifting for the sports featured in Chapter 11. Finally, I have a special recognition for Jeff Wittmer and Pat Hayes, the lifters who served as models for the bulk of the instructional technique shots.

Weightlifting is a fun, challenging, life-long activity. I trust *Explosive Lifting for Sports* will provide many with the opportunity and direction to maximize their potential.

Introduction

Sport in the 21st century has evolved to a higher level of performance than ever imagined by our predecessors. Sport performance today is a result of many variables, not the least of which is greatly improved strength and conditioning programs. The creation of a stronger, faster, more powerful body is the priority of most athletes and coaches.

Strength training is an accepted part of training for most sports. In a quest to use the *best* form of strength training, coaches and sport scientists have closely examined the sport of weightlifting. After all, weightlifters are among the strongest, most powerful athletes in the sporting world. However, weightlifting is a complicated sport that requires an understanding of the finer points before you can safely and effectively apply this type of training in your conditioning program.

Explosive Lifting for Sports is written for athletes, coaches, sport scientists, students, and fitness professionals who want to understand the subtle nuances of the sport, the lifts, and related training. Through a better understanding of how and why weightlifting movements are performed, you'll be ready to safely and effectively incorporate this training into your workouts.

This introduction explains specific terminology associated with weightlifting and other forms of strength training, along with the rationale for using explosive lifting for improved sport performance. Chapters 1 through 3 discuss the roles of strength, power, and plyometric training and the importance of these aspects in the creation of a more powerful athlete. Chapters 4 through 7 take the reader through a safe and effective learning sequence for the "classic" lifts used by weightlifters. Chapters 8 and 9 cover the proper execution of assistance exercises (also explosive in nature). Finally, chapters 10 and 11 address the basics of training programs and the actual use of explosive lifts for a variety of sports.

You won't find any in-depth explanation of explosive lifting elsewhere. The community of weightlifters and their coaches is pretty small. Most strength training books, if they cover explosive lifting at all, offer only a very brief explanation, which can be more dangerous than none at all. These lifts must be taught, learned, and executed properly in order to improve performance safely and effectively. Although an aspiring weightlifter will benefit greatly from reading *Explosive Lifting for Sports*, the book was written for the average athlete or coach wanting to incorporate the lifts into a strength training program.

The Sport of Weightlifting

Weightlifting, a competitive sport that has been part of the modern Olympic Games since 1896, addresses one of our most basic competitive urges:

the demonstration of strength. Although the sport has undergone numerous changes since its first days as an organized competition, weightlifting remains true to its original roots. The question How much can you lift? remains relevant today, even as demands for physical strength in 21st-century daily life have certainly been reduced.

Despite the reduced need for physical strength in most walks of life today, the use of resistance training for improved physical fitness is at an all-time high. Why this recent growth in popularity? After years of fighting for public acceptance, nearly all audiences realize that lifting weights offers many varied benefits, including the following:

- Increased strength and power for improved sport performance
- Improved muscular development and body composition
- Injury prevention or rehabilitation
- Improved health
- An opportunity to participate in competition

As physical fitness has become a more popular free-time activity, so has the manner in which people go about "lifting weights." It can be downright confusing for the newcomer to wade through all of the information offered on this subject. One of the primary purposes of this book is to clarify the terminology associated with "lifting weights" and to focus clearly on the origin of them all, the sport of weightlifting. This book was not meant to entice newcomers to the sport of weightlifting, although anyone wishing to get a start in this direction will certainly learn the basics of style and technique. Weightlifting techniques will help you maximize the benefits of resistance training, particularly for sports involving strength and power. By incorporating the secrets of weightlifting training offered in this book into your training program, you will be a better performer in nearly any sport.

We no longer have to do battle with "old wives' tales" about the negative consequences of resistance training. Lifting weights is widely accepted by nearly all coaches, athletes, medical professionals, sport scientists, and the general public. Even more widely accepted, particularly in athletic circles, is the use of weightlifting movements and training for the ultimate goal, improved athletic performance in sports requiring powerful muscular actions.

Terminology

Weightlifting (one word) refers to the competitive sport of lifting barbells as practiced in the Olympic Games. Both male and female competitors in different weight categories demonstrate their strength in two lifts that require the barbell to be hoisted overhead. The first lift is the *snatch*, in which the barbell is quickly pulled from the ground to arms' length overhead in one continuous motion. The second lift, the *clean-and-jerk*, is a two-part lift that consists of pulling the barbell from a starting position on the floor to the shoulders (the *clean*), and then after a brief recovery, thrusting the bar overhead by a combined effort of the legs and arms (the *jerk*).

Powerlifting is a competitive sport that evolved from weightlifting in the United States in the 1960s. It consists of three barbell lifts (squat, bench press, deadlift). This sport is not included in the Olympic Games.

Bodybuilding (or *physique*) is an activity that falls outside the normal sport performance arena. Bodybuilders do not compete by lifting barbells, although they do train with resistance methods and equipment. Bodybuilders simply display their muscularity to a panel of judges who subjectively decide the winner.

Weight training is the term used when someone lifts weights for the general purposes of improved health, sport performance, or physical appearance quests not as extreme as those of bodybuilders.

Strength training, a relatively new term, is applied to athletes who use resistance training to increase strength with the express purpose of improving performance in their chosen sport. Strength training implies that the athlete is actually using a high enough resistance, applied with a relatively low number of repetitions, to actually gain strength. Not everyone engaged in resistance training actually trains for increased strength.

Resistance training is the overall scientifically correct term for all of the previously mentioned forms of training. Resistance training implies the use of some form of external resistance, be it a barbell or dumbbells (free weights), resistance training machines, body weight, elastic tubing, or other forms of resistance applied for any one of the reasons listed earlier.

Resistance Training for Improved Athletic Performance

Until about 1960, athletes from other sports generally shunned the idea of lifting weights for improved athletic performance. For the most part, runners ran, swimmers swam, divers dove, and that was it. With the passage of time, the idea of athletes using resistance training to increase their performance on the field or court gradually took hold. This was a very slow process, as conventional wisdom at the time suggested that weightlifting or general weight training would cause numerous physical complications that would impair performance. Prominent figures in the physical education field, along with nonbelieving coaches, suggested that lifting weights would make players "muscle-bound," an expression that was never completely defined. Many assumed that if muscles got larger, players would not be able to move swiftly or with agility. Athletes and coaches feared that lifting weights would actually cause the athlete to become slower.

This argument continued for many years and in some isolated cases continues today. Among the first to slowly accept resistance training were football coaches who quickly noticed that those who trained with weights were bigger, faster, and stronger. Gradually, coaches and athletes in other sports came to embrace the use of resistance training for improved performance. While some holdouts still think that lifting weights will cause undue weight gain or excessive muscular growth, these people are becoming increasingly rare.

Today coaches and athletes generally believe that resistance training creates a stronger, faster player who will be more resistant to injury caused either by continuous practice of the sport or actual contact while engaged in the sport. But, while the concept has been nearly universally accepted, the details of how to best improve performance remain somewhat controversial.

What Type of Training Is Best?

Here the debate heats up considerably. Among those who embrace resistance training, there remain large and divergent camps as to how best to train. Some of this divisiveness is a result of how these proponents themselves trained as athletes. Those with a weightlifting background prefer the so-called explosive lifts (the snatch, clean, and jerk). Powerlifters encourage the use of heavy loads in the squat, bench press, and deadlift, without much concern for speed. Bodybuilders focus more on muscular development of many small-muscle groups that may or may not contribute to improved performance. To a certain extent this personal preference is understandable.

Another major contribution to the current debate appeared about 1970, with the introduction into the marketplace of more elaborate resistance training machines. In an attempt to convince athletes that *theirs* was the preferred means of training, manufacturers made many claims. These claims, many without qualitative or quantitative research to back them up, became suspect as a means of simply marketing the new machines.

This debate spurred the growth of a group that to date had been small and relatively silent: sport scientists. The growth of sport science in the past 20 years has been nothing short of phenomenal. As these experts took on the task of researching methods of training and how well they worked, however, the split opinions remained.

As we begin the 21st century, debate on the most efficient manner to apply resistance training focuses on several key topics: sport specific versus nonsport-specific training, free weights versus machines, and single sets versus multiple sets.

Sport-Specific Versus Nonsport-Specific Resistance Training

The term *sport-specific training* implies that exercises should mimic as much as possible the actions of the body during a given sport. This can mean exercising the body's joints and muscles through a range of motion similar to that used in the chosen sport and/or training the body's energy systems as they will be used in the chosen sport.

Sport science tells us that a boxer, who performs in repeated three-minute bouts with one minute of rest between, should train the body's energy system in a similar manner, such as by using interval training as opposed to long, slow distance runs. Likewise, a basketball player does not need to run endless laps around the court but should practice repeated short bursts of speed training and jumping. Despite the wisdom of sport science, however, old-school tradition often wins out.

Among strength and conditioning coaches there is nearly total acceptance of the notion of sport-specific training. We recognize that the *most* specific form of training is the actual performance of the chosen sport. But performing only the sport fails to provide the muscular overload needed to gain additional strength or power. Also, muscular imbalances may occur as a result of only performing a specific sport and not preparing the total body.

Total-body exercises performed explosively (the snatch, clean, and jerk) are considered a close approximation of the joint actions experienced by many athletes, especially those who depend on horizontal or vertical action (football players, basketball players, volleyball players, sprinters, weight throwers, etc.). The lifts are therefore called sport specific.

Opponents of explosive or weightlifting training often claim that these lifts bring an increased risk of injury. It is important to note that these lifts are not inherently dangerous; however, unqualified or inadequate coaching can certainly lead to injury, regardless of the exercise selected. Opponents similarly argue that a football lineman is never going to lift a barbell at the snap. This is true, but proponents claim that lifting a barbell from the platform requires the use of joint angles (ankle, knee, and hip) that are similar to those used in the lineman's starting position.

Opponents of explosive lifting often advocate seeking strength gains through nonspecific methods (particularly machines) and then converting those strength gains to useful, sport-specific actions by practicing the chosen sport.

One conclusion (perhaps the only sure one) is that either type of resistance training is better than none at all. Much of the debate depends on what sport is under discussion and how safely sport-specific movements can be performed with either machines or free weights.

For example, I assisted USA Cycling for many years with their strength training, due in part to my experience as a competitive cyclist and weightlifter. After looking at a cyclist's pedal stroke and the muscles (hip and knee extensors) involved, I had no trouble telling a cyclist that she would benefit more from squats than leg extensions. Unfortunately, one coach advised junior cyclists to perform squats with their feet staggered fore and aft about the same distance apart as bicycle pedals. Although this appeared to be quite sport specific, a squat cannot be performed safely in this position. Further, with the already better-than-average leg strength most cyclists possess, the weights used were relatively heavy. Squatting in such an awkward position was asking for trouble. This is an example of taking sport-specific training too far.

Free Weights Versus Resistance Machines

In terms of duplicating specific joint angles and motor pathways, free weights allow for many more sport-specific exercises than do machines. Free weights also usually allow for more precise incremental weight increases than do machines. Lifting free weights generally duplicates day-to-day activities much more closely. One of the biggest advantages of free weights is that your balance is challenged, just as in most sports.

In this age of ever more sophisticated technology we often look to machines or gadgets to provide an easier way to perform our work, including the work of exercise. Making training easier, however, may not produce the benefits we seek. Unfortunately, some machine manufacturers, in an attempt to "one-up" their competition, go to great lengths to create marketing ploys based on questionable science. While I've never seen a barbell company try to sell the advantages of free weights over machines, I have seen numerous machine companies take a swipe at this "stone age" approach to training while lauding their "space age" technology.

Single Sets Versus Multiple Sets

A set is a unit of repetitions performed continuously. Nearly everyone who uses free weights and sport-specific training methods will opt for multiple sets. Despite this, numerous studies have asserted that a single set of each exercise *nearly* matches the gains of multiple-set protocols. Many of these studies used untrained subjects in their experiments. There is little doubt that in short-term (up to 12 weeks or so) resistance training with novices, a single set does come close to equaling what is achieved with multiple sets. However, since most competitive athletes are *not* untrained subjects, the conclusions reached in these studies may not apply to them. Additionally, experiments carried out for a longer period (up to nine months) clearly indicate the superiority of multiple sets.

In any case, who wants to get *nearly* the same results? Certainly not many competitive athletes I've known. True enough, someone strapped for time who seeks only minimal muscular fitness gains can get by, in the short term, by performing only one set of each exercise.

Advantages of Weightlifting

Learned properly, explosive weightlifting movements should contribute to improved sport performance. The primary goal of *Explosive Lifting for Sports* is to teach safely and methodically the proper sequences for performing explosive lifts. The snatch, clean, and jerk, properly performed with today's technique, have been described as "jumping with weights." This powerful and coordinated effort can be of great assistance to athletes of many sports. A great deal of research has found a high correlation between proficient execution of the classic lifts (the snatch, clean, and jerk) and the vertical jump test. The vertical jump test is widely used to measure power, or explosiveness, a vital component of many athletic events.

Again, those who argue against the use of weightlifting training for athletes in other sports focus on either the possibility of injury or what they consider a lack of focus on sport-specific skills. I repeat the earlier message: There is nothing inherently dangerous about the snatch or clean-and-jerk lifts. Training injuries can occur under all sorts of conditions, including using resistance training machines. The key to avoiding injury is to know *how* to perform movements and do so in a professionally supervised setting.

Mastery of weightlifting is within nearly everyone's grasp, but as with any technical skill, it takes a great deal of practice. There is little doubt that learning a total-body exercise is more difficult than simply sitting on a machine and performing a relatively easy exercise such as an arm curl or a chest press. A resistance machine restricts you from doing anything it was not designed to do. A barbell, on the other hand, requires constant attention, focus, and feedback.

If your sport activity does not involve the entire body (such as in archery, paddling, or sailing), you may be better off with a simpler form of resistance training, such as resistance machines or simpler single-joint exercises. But fear should not be a reason for avoiding classic lifts. As is true of any exercise or athletic movement, those who do not know what they are doing or cannot demonstrate proper technique should not be performing the activity.

The lifts described in this book are not difficult to learn. This is particularly true of the noncompetitive movements such as the power snatch, the power clean, various pulling motions related to either of those lifts, the push press, the power jerk, or similar movements.

Males and females of all ages can master the classic lifts and the assistance exercises. Youngsters are quick to learn these lifts. Grandparents in their 70s and 80s regularly compete in masters' competitions. Weightlifting is a lifelong sport, enjoyable to all. If you want to take up weightlifting, there isn't much to hold you back.

If you don't want to become a weightlifter, simply use these lifts to improve your sport performance. If you aren't actively involved in a sport or if you are a personal trainer working with both athletic and nonathletic clientele, the use of these lifts for noncompetitive means introduces a challenging, fun way to improve fitness.

Athletes from many sports successfully train on the two competitive lifts or variations of them. As you'll see later in this book, many top coaches of sports such as football, basketball, and volleyball are very positive about the benefits derived from explosive training using weightlifting movements. Their players have benefited from snatch and clean-and-jerk training—perhaps not the full, competitive lifts but variations executed with lighter weights focused on developing power for their sport.

Due to the dynamic, total-body nature of these lifts, anyone practicing them is likely to exert more physical effort with a snatch or clean than with a curl or lat pull-down. Engaging the entire body in a successful performance takes more concentration and effort and as such results in a great expenditure of energy (calories). Heart rate and breathing both are at higher rates when performing these lifts than they are when performing exercises from a seated or prone position.

Personal trainers, whether they work with athletes or nonathletes, always look for new ways to stimulate interest in and challenge their clientele. Trainers can easily learn these techniques and use these lifts for a new, different, and highly effective form of training. Except in very rare instances, the snatch and clean-and-jerk lifts or their variations can be safely and effectively performed by anyone engaged in resistance training.

Before we start on the specifics of technique, however, let's look at the science behind the concept of using weightlifting exercises for improved sport performance.

Training for Optimal Strength

Strength is a key component of success in many sports. However, as we discussed in the introduction, just adding resistance training does not guarantee improved strength. Many athletes who engage in resistance training with elastic tubing, aquatic training, body weight, or even light to moderate weights fail to produce actual gains in strength. They may receive other benefits, such as injury prevention, but this type of training has limited benefits in terms of strength development.

Why some forms of resistance training may not produce gains in strength becomes clear when we define the term *strength*. Although the definition of *strength* is often debated, for our purposes strength is the ability to exert a maximal force against a resistance. Strength gains are fairly easily achieved with the appropriate use of resistance training of a sufficiently high intensity to elicit a strength response. Actual gains in strength normally require the use of either free weights or resistance machines.

Another important ingredient for success in many sports is power. Power is the subject of the following chapter, but for right now, keep in mind that power is the product of strength *and* speed. So, our discussion in this chapter about strength is crucial to the next step, improved power.

Let's look at what strength is and the characteristics of a training program designed to improve strength.

Types of Strength

The term *strength* is often linked to other words to describe a particular type of strength (speed strength, explosive strength, isometric strength). Rather than explore further the many scientific avenues associated with strength research, we will contain our discussion of strength to the basics. However, it is important to recognize two different types of, or ways to evaluate, strength: absolute strength and relative strength.

Absolute strength is synonymous with maximum muscular strength. Absolute strength is also low-speed strength, as in the sport of powerlifting, in which the lifts are not performed quickly because of the nature of the lifts and the massive weights that must be moved a good distance. Absolute strength improvement is crucial to many sports, particularly those that involve moving a heavy resistance (football, wrestling, weightlifting, powerlifting). Most sports, however, do not allow for such slow execution of movement.

It is important to know how crucial strength is for your sport and where you currently fit in that sport's strength continuum. More on this later.

The other form of strength that is important to address is *relative strength*. Relative strength is easily defined as your strength-to-weight ratio. How strong are you when strength is expressed as a percentage of your body weight? As we'll see later, male weightlifters have lifted more than three times their body weight overhead in the clean-and-jerk lift. Women have succeeded with more than twice their body weight. Contrary to powerlifters, weightlifters must execute their movements with blinding speed or they will simply lose the battle to gravity.

As you may imagine, lighter lifters have a better chance of lifting a higher percentage of their body weight than those at the higher end of the body weight continuum. Regardless of the lift, an athlete weighing 150 pounds (68 kilograms) has a better chance of lifting 150 to 450 pounds (68 to 204 kilograms) than an athlete weighing 250 pounds (113 kilograms) has with 250 to 750 pounds (113 to 340 kilograms). This is a simple matter of geometric progression.

Of course, other factors being equal, a larger athlete normally performs better in terms of absolute strength. This is why weightlifting has different body weight categories for lifters ranging from around 100 pounds to well over 300 pounds (45 to 136 kilograms).

Smaller individuals, on the other hand, generally display more relative strength. It is impossible to predict exactly the optimal strength-to-weight ratio of every athlete in every sport. As a result, some experimentation is needed to determine the proper body weight and body composition that will produce the best athletic performance.

Importance of Acceleration

In sports involving quick movements, the ability to accelerate a weight, or mass, is the key to success. This may involve only your own body weight with no additional resistance, as in a soccer player covering enough ground quickly to score. It may involve your body weight plus a light implement such as a tennis racket, as in a tennis player moving quickly enough to return an opponent's serve. It may mean your own body weight plus the mass of an opponent, such as in football or wrestling. In weightlifting, the opponent is the barbell.

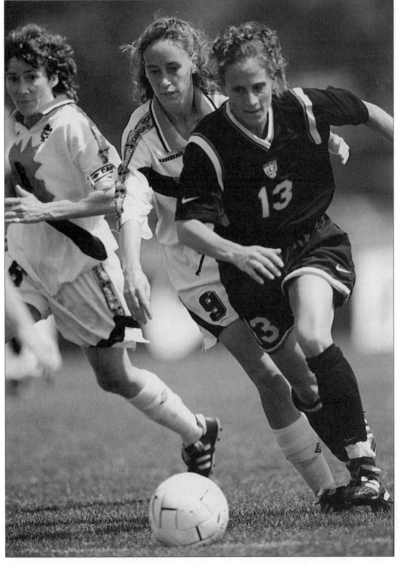

Explosive lifting improves acceleration, a trait needed for sports like soccer.

Newton's (unfortunately, no relation) Second Law of Motion deals with acceleration. It states that for bodies of constant mass, acceleration is proportional to the force that causes it and takes place in the direction in which the force acts. The relevant formula is $F = ma$, where F equals the amount of force available, m represents the mass involved, and a is the amount of acceleration available to move the mass.

You represent a certain mass, and any object you may attempt to lift also represents a mass. To move an object's mass successfully (either your own or your own with an opponent), you must exert an amount of force greater than that of the object. You can easily see that increasing your strength has a positive effect on the amount of force you can exert. The amount of time involved in your specific sport's movement (the rate of force production) dictates to a certain extent how beneficial increases in strength will be. In other words, it becomes very important to address the question How much stronger do I need to become to improve my sport performance by X amount?

Gaining strength improves your ability to accelerate a mass, provided you specifically train your acceleration skills as well. We'll talk later about simply using resistance training to gain strength, then using sport-specific training and competition experiences to sharpen athletic skills. The focal point of this book, explosive lifting, takes this concept one step further. By performing explosive lifts, not only do you get stronger (and faster) but you also improve your ability to accelerate against a progressively heavier mass.

Strength Gains and Body Weight

As we look at relative strength (which is generally the goal of strength training for most sports), what is the impact on your performance if you lose or gain weight? At what body weight and body composition do you show your best sport results? Depending on where you start, you may gain weight and improve relative strength not only in the weight room but also in your sport. For some, such a gain, while increasing relative strength, may not contribute to increased performance. Similarly, a loss of weight may or may not impact your relative strength, and it may or may not improve your sport performance.

Unfortunately, many athletes (particularly endurance types and far too many females) shy away from true strength training programs with high intensities and lower repetitions because they fear "bulking up." This rather vague expression means different things to different people, but in general, "bulking up" seems to be associated with increases in muscular size. The common, but unfounded, fear of many is that a gain in muscle size means an unneeded gain in body weight and a decrease in sport performance.

We know that gains in strength are related to intensity of effort. Using a high-intensity, low-repetition protocol maximizes strength gains, although it is unlikely to cause any significant gain in weight. It is also unlikely to maximize hypertrophy, or gains in muscular growth. Most athletes welcome gains in strength and power without a gain in size or weight.

Gains in body weight normally require an increased caloric intake or a reduced caloric expenditure (eat more or do less). Athletes training specifically for strength are unlikely to gain significant body weight unless they increase their food consumption or cut back on aerobic conditioning. Road cyclists often complained to me that they were gaining weight as a result of the resistance training they were performing during the off-season (October to February). Consider the fact that those who live where training is limited because of weather or little daylight training time in the off-season have considerably reduced activity levels in the off-season than they have in the summer months. Combine this with the likelihood of some additional eating near the holidays, and a weight gain may occur. However, it's not because of strength or resistance training.

Correct Amount of Strength

Strength and conditioning professionals continually examine the topic of the development of *appropriate* amounts of strength for a particular sport. Some athletes, particularly those with little need to display maximum, or absolute, strength in their game, waste time in the gym developing more strength than they can effectively use in their chosen sport. While this may do them no real harm, it is extra time and effort that could be used more appropriately elsewhere, such as training for their sport.

Since true strength development requires a high intensity, some athletes and coaches are concerned about a possible increase in injuries from heavy training. Some years ago, the top sprint cyclist in the United States met with me to discuss his strength training program. Here was a very gifted athlete who reportedly squatted 205 kilograms (451 pounds) for 10 repetitions (reps) and 250 kilograms (550 pounds) for 1 rep. He wanted to raise these figures to 227.5 kilograms (501 pounds) for 10 reps and 272.5 kilograms (600 pounds) for 1 rep. Having known and worked with this cyclist over several years, it was my impression that his lower body was physically prepared to achieve these goals. However, I was not convinced that his torso strength was adequate to support the desired load.

I've worked with enough elite athletes to know that it can be difficult to talk them out of certain goals, particularly those related to specific numbers. Thinking that I could not dissuade him from going after these goals, I asked about his torso training. He informed me that he performed back extensions, in sets of 20 repetitions, but with no resistance. Similarly, he routinely included abdominal "crunches" in his workout but, again, with high repetitions and only with body weight resistance. In other words, this part of his body was not engaged in true strength training. And, he related that his back had been occasionally injured, either as a result of crashes on the track or in the weight room.

This struck me as an accident waiting to happen. A load of 600 pounds resting on the shoulders must be supported by an extremely strong core musculature (abdominal, lower back, hip, and shoulder muscles). Would the additional squat performance have translated to a faster sprint? In other words, did he need to get stronger to go faster?

This sprinter regularly turned in the fastest qualifying times at world and Olympic competitions. He was probably already stronger than his competitors, and he was already the fastest cyclist on the track, when racing against the clock. According to his coaches, he would gain the most by improving his tactics. I decided that the best advice I could offer was that he should strengthen his torso with the use of more resistance in his standard exercises. I added that he did not need to become obsessed with certain numerical goals.

Within a year the nagging little "micro-injuries" to his back had added up, and he required surgery. Although I don't know the exact details or cause, I can safely say the pursuit of excessive strength beyond his needs probably contributed to this result. You want to develop *appropriate* strength for your sport. Anything beyond this may well be wasted effort and put you at risk for an unnecessary injury. Injuries in the weight room should not occur in athletes who only use resistance training as an adjunct for their primary sport.

No hard-and-fast rules exist for how much strength is appropriate. In many cases, normative data on athletes by gender and sport position are available. It can be useful to know where you rank with others in your sport. Deficiencies in strength-related measures may indicate that more strength training is needed, but this is a topic with no definite answer. If you determine that you need additional strength in a particular muscle area or performance measure, turn your attention to how to train specially for this gain in strength.

Muscles and Strength Testing

How the body's muscular system works and how this impacts sport performance is a fascinating topic. Complete texts are devoted to the topic of muscle physiology. While it is not within the scope of this book to address the topic in depth, some basic points of consideration are necessary.

Muscle Action

The actual measure of strength and strength gains is broken down into a series of muscle actions. *Concentric* muscle action occurs when a muscle or set of muscles shortens against resistance. In the classic example of an arm curl, the elbow joint flexes to elevate a barbell or dumbbell. This requires the elbow flexors to shorten or contract until the resistance is raised to its final position near the collarbones, where the joint is fully closed.

Eccentric muscle action occurs when a muscle or group of muscles lengthens against resistance. In our curl example, this is the lowering of the weight from the collarbones to the starting position. The same muscle group has gone through both concentric and eccentric muscle actions to perform one repetition. Some people get confused and think that eccentric action somehow relates to the elbow extensors, the triceps. This muscle group is not a prime mover in the arm curl, so neither muscle action is attributed to it. Eccentric muscle action normally allows for loads larger than those allowed by concentric muscle action.

Isometric muscle action occurs when no movement happens around a joint; rather, muscles simply perform a static hold against an object. Sports such as archery, shooting, and wrestling require isometric muscle action.

Strength Testing

A great deal of research has been conducted to determine safe and effective ways to test maximal strength. Remember that strength is the ability to exert *maximal* force. The old standby test for strength is the 1-RM, or 1 repetition maximum, test in a prescribed exercise. 1-RM intensity means that you are successful with one rep but fail when attempting a second rep. If you succeed with a second rep, this resistance is your 2-RM; you will need more weight to perform a 1-RM.

"Maxing out" with free weights, especially for a novice or a nonpower athlete, may be dangerous because of an athlete's unfamiliarity with making this type of effort in an unfamiliar lift. If this novice first goes through a training period to learn how to perform the lift at such a high level of intensity, thus improving his safety, such training will positively bias the resulting test performance.

In an attempt to avoid the problems associated with performing a 1-RM test, some coaches and sport scientists use a multiple-repetition performance with weights and estimate what the 1-RM should be (see table 1.1). For example, approximately 130 percent of a subject's 10-RM is the estimated 1-RM in many exercises. Squats with 200 pounds (91 kilograms) for 10 reps (when the athlete is not capable of performing an 11th rep) would result in an estimated 1-RM of 260 pounds (118 kilograms). This is not extremely accurate and may vary widely based on the athlete's experience and the lift in question. And of course, a novice performing a true 10-RM may be in some danger of injury as well.

Many sources suggest the use of body weight resistance in numerous calisthenic-type exercises to safely test for strength. The problem with using higher repetitions (15 or more) in such exercises as push-ups, pull-ups, or abdominal curls, as we'll see later on, is that we get more of a measure of muscular endurance than muscular strength.

A number of fitness equipment manufacturers have introduced various machines to the market that purport to measure strength in a safe and controlled manner, but such machines introduce further complications, such as mechanical advantage.

One of the big hurdles with strength testing is that many of the lifts that safely measure strength of a certain set of muscles have nothing to do with functional, or everyday, movements, to say nothing of sport-specific movements. So, while the industry continues to battle with this dilemma, the 1-RM test, despite numerous drawbacks, can be considered a valid test of strength, at least for the muscles involved and for that particular lift. Sport-specific strength training for many movements, especially those that involve the element of speed for execution, is still to be developed.

Developing Strength

True strength training requires a high resistance to actually produce gains in strength. Simply lifting weights or making use of resistance machines or other forms of resistance will not guarantee that you'll get stronger. Gains in strength require attention to a certain number of variables.

TABLE 1.1

Estimating 1-RM and Training Loads

Max reps (RM)	1	2	3	4	5	6	7	8	9	10	12	15
%1-RM	100	95	93	90	87	85	83	80	77	75	67	65
Load (lb or kg)	10	10	9	9	9	9	8	8	8	8	7	7
	20	19	19	18	17	17	17	16	15	15	13	13
	30	29	28	27	26	26	25	24	23	23	20	20
	40	38	37	36	35	34	33	32	31	30	27	26
	50	48	47	45	44	43	42	40	39	38	34	33
	60	57	56	54	52	51	50	48	46	45	40	39
	70	67	65	63	61	60	58	56	54	53	47	46
	80	76	74	72	70	68	66	64	62	60	54	52
	90	86	84	81	78	77	75	72	69	68	60	59
	100	95	93	90	87	85	83	80	77	75	67	65
	110	105	102	99	96	94	91	88	85	83	74	72
	120	114	112	108	104	102	100	96	92	90	80	78
	130	124	121	117	113	111	108	104	100	98	87	85
	140	133	130	126	122	119	116	112	108	105	94	91
	150	143	140	135	131	158	125	120	116	113	101	98
	160	152	149	144	139	136	133	128	123	120	107	104
	170	162	158	153	148	145	141	136	131	128	114	111
	180	171	167	162	157	153	149	144	139	135	121	117
	190	181	177	171	165	162	158	152	146	143	127	124
	200	190	186	180	174	170	166	160	154	150	134	130
	210	200	195	189	183	179	174	168	162	158	141	137
	220	209	205	198	191	187	183	176	169	165	147	143
	230	219	214	207	200	196	191	184	177	173	154	150
	240	228	223	216	209	204	199	192	185	180	161	156
	250	238	233	225	218	213	208	200	193	188	168	163
	260	247	242	234	226	221	206	208	200	195	174	169
	270	257	251	243	235	230	224	216	208	203	181	176
	280	266	260	252	244	238	232	224	216	210	188	182
	290	276	270	261	252	247	241	232	223	218	194	189

Max reps (RM)	1	2	3	4	5	6	7	8	9	10	12	15
%1-RM	100	95	93	90	87	85	83	80	77	75	67	65
Load (lb or kg)	300	285	279	270	261	255	249	240	231	225	201	195
	310	295	288	279	270	264	257	248	239	233	208	202
	320	304	298	288	278	272	266	256	246	240	214	208
	330	314	307	297	287	281	274	264	254	248	221	215
	340	323	316	306	296	289	282	272	262	255	228	221
	350	333	326	315	305	298	291	280	270	263	235	228
	360	342	335	324	313	306	299	288	277	270	241	234
	370	352	344	333	322	315	307	296	285	278	248	241
	380	361	353	342	331	323	315	304	293	285	255	247
	390	371	363	351	339	332	324	312	300	293	261	254
	400	380	372	360	348	340	332	320	308	300	268	260
	410	390	381	369	357	349	340	328	316	308	274	267
	420	399	391	378	365	357	349	336	323	315	281	273
	430	409	400	387	374	366	357	344	331	323	288	280
	440	418	409	396	383	374	365	352	339	330	295	286
	450	428	419	405	392	383	374	360	347	338	302	293
	460	437	428	414	400	391	382	368	354	345	308	299
	470	447	437	423	409	400	390	376	362	353	315	306
	480	456	446	432	418	408	398	384	370	360	322	312
	490	466	456	441	426	417	407	392	377	368	328	319
	500	475	465	450	435	425	415	400	385	375	335	325
	510	485	474	459	444	434	423	408	393	383	342	332
	520	494	484	468	452	442	432	416	400	390	348	338
	530	504	493	477	461	451	440	424	408	398	355	345
	540	513	502	486	470	459	448	432	416	405	362	351
	550	523	512	495	479	468	457	440	424	413	369	358
	560	532	521	504	487	476	465	448	431	420	375	364
	570	542	530	513	496	485	473	456	439	428	382	371
	580	551	539	522	505	493	481	464	447	435	389	377
	590	561	549	531	513	502	490	472	454	443	395	384
	600	570	558	540	522	510	498	480	462	450	402	390

Reprinted, by permission, from Baechle, Earle, and Wathen, 2000, "Resistance Training." In *Essentials of strength training and conditioning*, edited by Baechle and Earle (Champaign, IL: Human Kinetics), 410–411.

Theory of Progressive Resistance

To make continued gains in strength, you need to use a progressive overload. The theory of progressive resistance, which relates to all aspects of physical conditioning, not just resistance training, states that you must periodically make the effort more difficult in order to coax the muscles to a higher level of response. Failure to do so results in your previous effort becoming submaximal, which will prevent you from getting stronger.

But what if you are not interested in becoming a strength/power athlete? How important is maximal strength in your sport, and would increased strength translate to improved performance? The answers vary greatly depending on the sport in question. As mentioned earlier, if your sport requires moving a relatively heavy object (as in football or wrestling), strength is a primary concern and a fair amount of your training should be devoted to developing strength and power. If your sport requires use of a smaller resistance (as in basketball, tennis, or volleyball), absolute strength is not quite as important. Power is the key to your continued success. But as we will discuss in the next chapter, power generally improves as a result of increased strength.

Channel absolute strength into power and see the benefits on the basketball court.

Repetitions Determine Strength Gain

Weightlifters, powerlifters, and bodybuilders all lift weights. However, there is very little crossover or transfer of skills among these disciplines. This may be due to the genetic differences in the athletes attracted to each discipline or to the effects of different styles of training.

Many athletes from a myriad of different sports engage in resistance training, yet their individual results vary considerably. The high jumper or tennis player who lifts to improve sport performance will most likely exhibit no skill at weightlifting, powerlifting, or bodybuilding. Nonathletes working out in the gym may not actually gain strength or hypertrophy for all their efforts. Why do people doing essentially the same activity obtain so many different results?

Early research indicated that the repetition scheme used in resistance training (and as a result, the resistance applied) dictates the type of benefit you will receive from such training. What was discovered years ago in terms of the amount of work (as measured by repetitions) is true today as well. A continuum of repetitions exists, and results are fairly specific to the type of training you perform. Figure 1.1 illustrates the general benefits associated with a particular range of repetitions.

Weightlifters and powerlifters primarily interested in exhibiting power and strength to move heavy resistance perform most of their training in the one to six rep range. In reality, most of their training occurs in the one to three rep range, although somewhat higher reps are applied at certain times of the year or in certain exercises. Repetitions beyond five are rarely performed.

Bodybuilders, concerned with muscular hypertrophy, work mostly in the 8 to 12 rep range. This higher rep scheme requires a more moderate load. Muscular growth is more likely to occur by training in this range because of the repetitions used. However, since bodybuilders rarely lift in the one to six rep range, they seldom exhibit the strength characteristics of weightlifters or powerlifters. True enough, bodybuilders are stronger than the average

RM	≤2	3	4	5	6	7	8	9	10	11	12	13	14	15	16	17	18	19	≥20
Training goal		Strength					Strength					Strength				Strength			
		Power					Power					Power				Power			
		Hypertrophy					Hypertrophy					Hypertrophy				Hypertrophy			
						Muscular endurance					Muscular endurance					Muscular endurance			

FIGURE 1.1   General benefits associated with repetition.

Reprinted, by permission, from Baechle, Earle, and Wathen, 2000, "Resistance Training." In *Essentials of strength training and conditioning*, edited by Baechle and Earle (Champaign, IL: Human Kinetics), 414.

person in the gym, but the results they gain from a moderate load and a moderate rep range produce more muscular growth than absolute strength.

Keep in mind that bodybuilders also follow extreme diets and focus on more exercises per body part than an athlete simply wishing to lift for improved sport performance. This 8 to 12 rep range should not result in the same extremes of muscular growth for the average person. Another characteristic of bodybuilding training is a relatively short recovery period between sets. This results in positive effects on cardiovascular fitness. By comparison, weightlifters and powerlifters often sit down between sets and take several minutes before returning to another high-intensity set.

Individuals who perform resistance training around 15 reps per set have as their priority muscular endurance. This means that the involved muscles continue to function against a relatively light resistance. As a result, almost no strength and only minimal hypertrophy gains are obtained. And for those who lift greater than 15 reps, the resistance is so light that no actual strength gain occurs. In addition, a significant hypertrophic effect is unlikely to occur.

In general, endurance athletes are better off using their preferred sport to obtain sport-specific muscular endurance training. Resistance training in the weight room is more appropriately focused on developing strength and power or preventing injury.

Varying Training Philosophies

In terms of repetitions, how you should train is fairly easy to determine. This depends largely on what you want to gain from resistance training. As we will discuss later in the book, anyone using resistance training benefits from the use of different types of rep/load schemes at different times of the year. This is not a seasonal phenomenon but a component of periodization, or the use of different volumes and intensities in your training. Later on we will discuss in greater detail something called the general adaptation syndrome, in which such training variety provides a different stimulus for the muscles, thus leading to further improvements.

Most people engaged in resistance training work in the 8 to 12 rep range. They may not develop the muscular hypertrophy of a bodybuilder, but this is the standard model of general training. Although their strength and power are not maximized, relative gains in strength may occur. In other words, if you start out using 150 pounds (68 kilograms) for 10 reps in the bench press and train for six months (following the theory of progressive resistance), your muscles will adapt to the load and you'll be strong enough to perhaps bench press 180 pounds (82 kilograms) for 10 reps. Your strength *appears* to have increased by 20 percent.

In reality, some of these gains, particularly during the first 12 or so weeks, are due to what we call *neural adaptation*. This means that your brain and body have learned how to successfully "fire" to achieve the goal of moving the resistance. Neural adaptations account for a large amount of early progress. True strength gains tend to come later.

In the previous example, had you chosen to train for strength, that is, you performed one to six reps with higher resistance, chances are that your bench press would have moved up a greater amount in six months. A comparison of your initial results versus those later on would more accurately reflect improvement in strength. Keep in mind, strength gains from training with moderate loads in the 8 to 12 repetition range tend to be less than those associated with higher intensities used in one to six rep protocols.

As we discussed in the introduction, experts in the strength and conditioning field disagree on how athletes should train to make optimal gains. This debate is basically divided into two camps: those who believe in explosive, power-oriented resistance training and those who do not.

The former group argues for what they consider to be sport-specific movements, in terms of similar joint angles and energy system duplication. They generally agree that explosive weightlifting movements are similar to numerous sport actions, and so they promote explosive weightlifting and other movements. They tend to recommend ballistic (explosive) training with free weights, weighted objects, and body weight resistance.

The second group discourages any use of ballistic movements. They instead promote a minimal amount of time in the weight room, with a low number of sets (perhaps as few as one), but each set is performed to temporary muscle fatigue at about 12 reps. Many followers of this group encourage the use of plate-loaded resistance machines, thus avoiding the use of barbells. They definitely discourage the use of any explosive movements, with or without a barbell.

This debate is an interesting one to follow, with zealots on both sides of the argument. It can be quite confusing for a neophyte coach or athlete to wade through the different opinions to determine what is best. Certainly any training is better than none at all. For some athletes, particularly those missing a ballistic component in their chosen sport, ballistic training may not be tremendously advantageous. I don't suggest that all athletes train explosively, but because of my extensive background in weightlifting, I recognize the benefits this type of training creates for many athletes.

Before the 1992 Olympics I was asked by USA Cycling to talk with a young Lance Armstrong about the benefits of plyometric training. Armstrong's forte was endurance cycling, and there was nothing to indicate that his genetic makeup favored explosive-type activities. Although I viewed plyometrics as having a possible role in improving his ability to move more ballistically on the bike, sport scientists at the U.S. Olympic Committee suggested that he not spend time training explosively. History has proven this advice to be sound, although I imagine that his sprint and vertical jump are still not particularly good. He succeeded by focusing on his strong points and not having his weak points get in the way of success.

Explosive Training for Increased Strength

Other things being equal, a more powerful weightlifter lacking absolute strength will very likely beat a stronger, less powerful lifter *at weightlifting or power-specific lifts*. This is due to the overall nature of the lifts involved. This is a fine balance, however, as it is not unusual to see a relatively weak lifter pull a weight to the chest in a squat clean but be unable to stand up with the load. This is an example of good power but insufficient strength. Such a lifter needs to strengthen her hips and quadriceps through more squatting and other strengthening exercises.

Training with weightlifting-specific methods offers a great blend of both strength and power. However, not even the finest weightlifters train only with weightlifting movements. Their training also includes a large amount of strength development exercises such as squats and pulling motions.

Measured by pure strength performance, weightlifters may not be the strongest athletes on the planet. They do demonstrate outstanding strength, but if placed in a powerlifting competition, the average weightlifter will come out behind the powerlifter. The opposite is true of the average powerlifter who attempts the sport of weightlifting. Keep in mind that it is difficult to compare these two sports, even in a standard exercise such as a squat, since powerlifters use a different technique and many equipment "props" to achieve their goal of lifting the most weight. Weightlifters squat to improve their performance on the two classic lifts.

This chapter explored the importance of strength in sport performance. While we know that resistance training easily improves your strength, the question remains: Will you benefit most from gains in strength, power, or a combination of both? To get closer to the answer, let's now look at power and its characteristics.

Developing Explosive Power

Coaches, athletes, and the general public sometimes misuse the term *power*. Quite often the concepts of power and strength are used interchangeably, but this is a mistake and can cause confusion as to how you should train for improved performance. Power is much more a measure of combined speed and strength. In fact, these are the two factors we normally address in attempting to improve an athlete's power.

In the introduction I mentioned the current debate surrounding the concept of sport-specific training. Everyone agrees that practicing your actual sport is the best form of sport-specific training. However, to only practice your sport (without any additional overload) may keep you from developing the additional strength and power needed for improved performance and injury prevention.

On one side of the argument is a group that claims that the *only* sport-specific training is practice and performance of the sport itself, perhaps with added resistance in order to gain strength. This group may or may not also include a general resistance program in their athletes' training.

On the other side of the argument is a group that claims that athletes should perform exercises in the gym that mimic the joint actions and speeds used in their sport. This group believes that sport-specific resistance training does not need to be identical to sport performance; rather, it need only duplicate the motions with resistance.

Athletes and coaches know that they must address power in order to get better, but details on how to accomplish this are sometimes overlooked. In order to help clarify some of the confusion surrounding this topic, let's start with a definition of power. Remembering our previous discussion on strength, we'll then cover training for power. This combination of training for strength and power creates the foundation for your use of explosive training for improved sport performance.

Defining Power

Scientifically, power is defined as the rate at which work is performed. We've discussed the fact that many sports require outstanding power for success. In football this may mean a lineman quickly moving an opponent aside. In athletics it may mean a high jumper launching her body up and over the bar. Power is also what a weightlifter needs to rapidly lift a heavy barbell overhead.

Other texts have devoted many pages to the scientific discussion and definition of power and its related parameters. In order to keep our focus practical, with an emphasis on usable knowledge related to appropriate resistance training, let's use a simple formula for power:

Power = work (mass × distance) ÷ time

Work is defined as the product of an object's *mass* (weight) times the *distance* the object is moved. Work is divided by the elapsed *time* involved, which produces a unit of power, measuring the rate at which work was performed. In weightlifting, this means the weight (mass) of the barbell, the distance the weight is raised (snatch to arms' length overhead, clean to the shoulders, jerk from the shoulders to arms' length overhead), and the amount of time required to complete the lift.

Confusion between the terms *power* and *strength* is evident when we consider the sport of powerlifting, mentioned briefly in the introduction. Originally referred to as the "odd-lifts" when competition began in the United States in the late 1950s and early 1960s, the sport was called "strength-lifting" by the British about the same time. This is the scientifically correct term for the activity. However, because of international politics, the sport was officially launched into the international arena with the misnomer of powerlifting.

Considering the definition of power, you see that powerlifting does not really involve a great deal of measured power. Compared with weightlifting, the powerlifts (squat, bench press, and deadlift) take longer to elevate a heavier weight a shorter distance. This results in a relatively low measure of power. You can easily see the difference in power in these two sports by looking at table 2.1, from noted sport scientist John Garhammer, PhD.

So, while powerlifting may not be the best way to train specifically for power, it is a good way to train for strength. And, depending on your sport and your own current physical abilities, both strength and power may be important.

To understand clearly and appreciate the difference between strength and power, let's look at what is called a force-velocity curve. Figure 2.1 illustrates that maximum force occurs when velocity is zero (isometric muscle action). Conversely, maximum velocity occurs with minimal resistance.

Factors Affecting Power

To produce power, you need both strength and speed. Fortunately, both of these ingredients can be increased through the use of appropriate and systematic training. Individual differences account for much of the variation in how different people respond to specific training. Some very strong genetic

TABLE 2.1

Power Output During Execution of Selected Lifts

Lift	Subject	Power (W)
Bench press	Novice (60%—2 RM) Novice (85%—2 RM) Novice (100%—2 RM) Light novice Light elite Heavy elite	481 366 247 243 267 415
Deadlift	(Similar to squat values)	
Squat	Heavy elite (93%) Heavy elite	1,259 900
Snatch	Light elite (95%) Light elite	2,821 2,675
Clean	Heavy elite (92%) Heavy elite	3,877 3,413

Note: All values are for 1-RM unless listed otherwise. Values are for a specific elite athlete for each lift except bench presses, which are group averages. All values, except bench presses, include horizontal work and work performed to elevate the body's center of gravity.

Reprinted, by permission, from John Garhammer, 1989, "Weight Lifting and Training." In *Biomechanics of sport*, edited by Christopher L. Vaughn (Boca Raton, FL: CRC Press, LLC), 187.

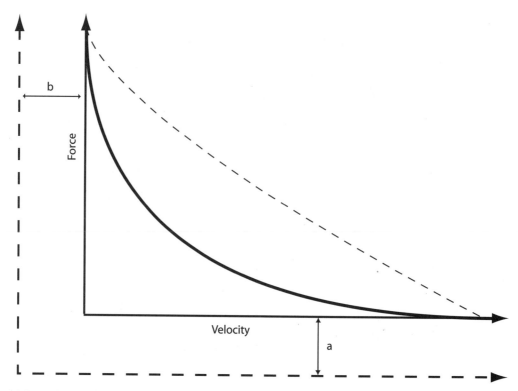

FIGURE 2.1 **The force-velocity curve illustrates the inverse relationship between maximum force and maximum velocity.**

factors are clearly associated with speed and power capabilities among individuals.

The most important genetic difference related to power development is the amount of muscle fiber that allows for quick muscular contraction. Your body's skeletal musculature is made up of several types of fibers. Type I fibers, the so-called slow-twitch (ST) muscle fibers, are associated with less powerful, more enduring functions. These fibers, being more aerobic in nature, take longer to develop force and to fatigue.

Type II muscle fibers, the so-called fast-twitch (FT) fibers, are associated with shorter bursts of explosive action. These fibers, which are used during anaerobic performance, develop force more quickly and fatigue more easily. Type II fibers are further subdivided into Type IIa and Type IIb fibers, with a-types having greater ability for aerobic metabolism and more resistance to fatigue.

The proportion and distribution of FT fibers throughout your body depends to a great extent on your genetic makeup. The average person has an approximate 50-50 split of FT and ST fibers throughout the body. Athletes who excel at power events tend to have a higher percentage of FT fibers, however, and those who excel at endurance events tend to have a higher percentage of ST fibers, compared to the average person.

That leaves many of us somewhere in the middle, perhaps not "natural" stars at either sprinting or long-distance events but capable of improving our performance in either extreme with specialized training. While you cannot do anything to alter the number of ST or FT fibers you were born with, stimulating the FT fibers you do have with explosive training improves their ability to fire or contract powerfully. This is the primary rationale for training for increased power: We *can* improve our FT fibers.

Determining Muscle Fiber Type

Knowing your genetic predisposition toward either aerobic or anaerobic sports can be an important consideration when choosing a sport. If you enjoy and excel at either endurance or power sports, you may already have a clue as to your muscle fiber composition. A long-distance runner enjoys running for hours and probably gravitates toward endurance events. He spends little, if any, time training sprints and does poorly in sprint events. On the flip side, a 50-meter freestyle swimmer spends nearly all her time devoted to rapid, short-distance training and can't stand endurance training.

If you like both long- and short-distance events but don't necessarily excel at one or the other, this may simply mean that one fiber type is not more dominant than the other. Sport scientists tell us that we can selectively train FT or ST fibers, just by the mode of training selected. But, to save time and effort, what if you want to know if you are genetically suited for one type of event over another? In this case we need to remove some of the guesswork and determine more accurately what percentage of ST and FT fibers you have.

Muscle Biopsy

The most objective way to determine your percentage of ST and FT fibers is to undergo a muscle biopsy. In this case, a small amount of muscle tissue is removed from the "belly" of the muscle (typically, the quadriceps). This is then stained for clear identification and examined under a microscope. An estimate of how many ST and FT cells are available is determined. While this method is quite accurate, it is beyond the means of the average athlete, unless you want to volunteer as a subject for a university human performance study. Besides, it takes a while to recover from having this tissue taken out of your thigh. How can the average athlete get an idea of his fiber typing without undergoing a biopsy?

Vertical Jump

Most athletes know from experience whether or not they excel at short-duration, explosive events, such as sprints. The vertical jump test is a good way to more objectively determine your ability in power events. While it won't tell you what percentage of FT fibers you have, it will help you determine the amount of explosiveness available.

The vertical jump test is easily administered and requires a minimum of equipment (figure 2.2). Stand at a right angle to a wall or chalkboard. Mark your right fingertips with chalk. Reach as high as possible and place your right hand on the surface. Lower your right arm and rechalk. With no steps and only a quick bend of the ankles, knees, and hips, dip down and explosively jump as high as possible, again marking the board at your maximum height from the floor. Record the distance between these two marks.

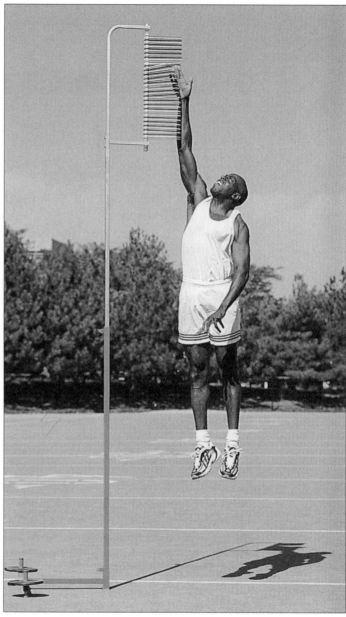

FIGURE 2.2   The vertical jump test is a standard measure of lower body power.

Reprinted, by permission, from Harman, Garhammer and Pandorf, 2000 "Administration, Scoring, and Interpretation of Selected Tests." In *Essentials of strength training and conditioning*, edited by Baechle and Earle (Champaign, IL: Human Kinetics), 293.

For sports that require vertical leaping (basketball or volleyball), this test is quite specific. For sports involved in horizontal movement (sprinting, football, shot put), the test is less specific but still an excellent measure of lower-body power. Table 2.2 will help you compare yourself to others in the vertical jump.

As we will see later in the book, successful execution of weightlifting movements amounts to jumping with additional weight in your hands. Those with good explosiveness in the vertical jump tend to transfer this skill to lifting the barbell. Those who do not jump particularly well can, nonetheless, improve their jumping ability, overall strength, and weightlifting-specific skills by practicing these lifts.

TABLE 2.2

Vertical Jump

Sport/position	Vertical jump in.	cm
NCAA Division I college football split ends, strong safetys, offensive and defensive backs	31.5	80
NCAA Division I college football wide receivers and outside linebackers	31	79
NCAA Division I college football linebackers, tight ends, safetys	29.5	75
College basketball players (men)	27-29	69-74
NCAA Division I college football quarterbacks	28.5	72
NCAA Division I college football defensive tackles	28	71
NCAA Division I college basketball players (men)	28	71
NCAA Division I college football offensive guards	27	69
Competitive college athletes (men)	25-25.5	64-65
NCAA Division I college football offensive tackles	25-26	64-66
Recreational college athletes (men)	24	61
High school football backs and receivers	24	61
College baseball players (men)	23	58
College tennis players (men)	23	58
High school football linebackers and tight ends	22	56
College football players	21	53
College basketball players (women)	21	53
17-year-old boys	20	51
High school football linemen	20	51
NCAA Division II college basketball guards (women)	19	48
NCAA Division II college basketball forwards (women)	18	46
NCAA Division II college basketball centers (women)	17.5	44
Sedentary college students (men)	16-20.5	41-52
18- to 34-year-old men	16	41
Competitive college athletes (women)	16-18.5	41-47
College tennis players (women)	15	38
Recreational college athletes (women)	15-15.5	38-39
Sedentary college students (women)	8-14	20-36
17-year-old girls	13	33
18- to 34-year-old women	8	20

The values listed are either means or 50th percentiles (medians). There was considerable variation in sample size among the groups tested. Thus, the data should be regarded as only descriptive, not normative.

Adapted, by permission, from Harman, Garhammer, and Pandorf, 2000. "Administration, Scoring, and Interpretation of Selected Tests." In *Essentials of strength training and conditioning*, edited by Baechle and Earle (Champaign, IL: Human Kinetics), 310.

Measuring Upper-Body Power

The seated medicine ball throw is among the most popular methods of measuring upper-body power.

Sit in a comfortable, upright chair, resting your back against the chair back. Bend your knees 90 degrees, and keep your feet flat on the floor. Truly objective testing calls for the torso to be secured to the back of the chair so as to cancel any upper-body motion. Alternatively, sit on the floor with your feet in front of you and your back against a wall. Take a weighted medicine ball and hold it with both hands directly in front of your sternum. Place your elbows away from your sides, in line with the forward thrust of the ball.

Take a breath, hold it momentarily, and push the medicine ball away from your chest as quickly as possible. Another individual records the spot where the medicine ball hits the floor. A third assistant is positioned directly behind the chair so that the forceful thrust does not cause you to tip over.

Although a popular test, finding results for your particular sport may require some research. Check first with a college strength coach, but be sure to confirm the weight of the medicine ball used.

Upper-body pulling power can also be measured using the standard pull-up. Hang at complete arms' length, then rapidly flex (bend) your elbows until your chin is above the bar. No known standards exist for this test, but an independent evaluator can easily count the number of repetitions you perform explosively, stopping your performance once the action no longer resembles a power movement but has become a slower strength or muscular endurance event.

Gaining Power

Most sports are ground based; that is, they are performed with the feet on the ground. Much of the power related to sport movement is generated in the lower body and the torso musculature. This force is then transferred to the extremities. (If your sport requires power in the torso and upper body, there are a number of ways to both test and train these parts as well.) If your vertical jump test indicated an above-average result, you may be genetically predetermined to do well in power-oriented sports.

If your results were not too outstanding, don't despair. A number of ways exist to train those FT fibers that you do have. A strong focus on training for explosive strength should create an increase in your vertical jump and other power measures, along with improving your ability to perform better at power events. Power is easily developed by training explosively with classic weightlifting exercises such as the snatch, the clean-and-jerk, and the related assistance movements.

Snatch or clean-and-jerk lifts cannot be performed slowly, unlike many other exercises that can be done either slowly or fast. Training for power with explosive lifts allows you to selectively stimulate your FT fibers and their rate of firing.

Slow resistance training, due either to a deliberately slow tempo of flexion and extension or a resistance so high you cannot move it quickly, does not specifically enhance power development. In the latter case, strength gains occur and added strength can contribute to improved power. But despite many claims to the contrary, a deliberately slow tempo of contraction requires a very light intensity. Such a light intensity does not provide an appropriate stimulus for increases in strength, power, or muscular growth.

If you perform your resistance training slowly, you'll need to focus on a great deal of sport-specific skill training in practice and competition in order to apply appropriately any additional strength gains created by your resistance training. Generally speaking, if you compete powerfully, you're better off resistance training explosively.

Power Training Benefits

A needs assessment review of your particular sport is important in order to know the physical qualities required, how to obtain these qualities most effectively, and when to focus on different types of training in order to peak at the right time. This needs assessment encompasses all fitness qualities: body composition, energy system fitness (aerobic vs. anaerobic needs), muscular fitness issues (absolute strength, power, muscular endurance), and flexibility.

Keep in mind that it is best for you to address each of these fitness issues, not just specialize in those qualities most prevalent in your sport. In other words, every athlete will benefit from training and improving each fitness characteristic, even if a specific characteristic does not contribute a great amount to sporting success. The proper balance depends on a sound, year-round training program that addresses different needs at different times of the year.

Power training is most beneficial at the beginning of your in-season phase of training. While power training should go on throughout the year, it becomes more of a priority toward the end of the preseason and beginning of the in-season. This allows for early season competitive results to reflect accurately the positive changes brought about during the off-season phase of training.

Skill Sports

With exceptions, athletes in *skill-oriented* sports that involve little movement (archery, bowling, shooting) probably do not require a particular emphasis on either strength or power. They will benefit from a more general resistance training program, which will help balance their overall musculature and aid in injury prevention.

There are always exceptions. One very enthusiastic athlete who used weightlifting-specific training was Ruby Fox, many times a champion pistol shooter. I learned of her attraction to these lifts when we were both on a Pan American Games team together. Why weightlifting for a shooter? Ruby felt that the total focus of having to execute the lift with split-second timing had a positive effect on her shooting. And, she gained overall strength and power benefits at the same time!

Skill and Agility Sports

Athletes involved in *skill and agility* sports (tennis, racquetball, soccer, ice hockey) may not need to perform exercises with high resistance since their sports do not involve heavy opposing resistance. They will benefit greatly from sport-specific agility drill work, both with and without additional resistance. These athletes may also benefit from training explosively in order to facilitate specific and/or nonspecific movement patterns and reaction times. Their actual sport practice then focuses on sport-specific speed and agility.

Improvements in power will result in more efficient sport-specific movement patterns, an ability to demonstrate powerful movements repetitively, and an overall resistance to injury caused by repetitive motions.

Many skill and agility sports also require rotational ability not addressed through conventional weightlifting or strength training. This requires a number of ground-based rotational exercises in order to improve this aspect of the musculature and to avoid injury.

Power for a tennis player, for instance, is likely to provide numerous benefits. Additional power in serving and returning strokes will be paramount to an improved game. Greater power will allow you to cover more territory quickly and increase your chances of returning your opponent's latest stroke. The added strength that is part of improved power, along with the actual training for improved power, will have a positive effect on your resistance to injury from overuse, repetitive motion, or multidirectional stresses to the body.

Strength Sports

Athletes involved in predominantly *strength* sports (powerlifting or the recent "strongman/woman" competitions) spend a greater percentage of their training on the powerlifts or other lifts without an emphasis on speed of execution. This may be a group that will benefit from slow training.

In reality, it's hard to find a popular mostly strength sport other than powerlifting. Wrist wrestling, tug-of-war, and so forth are all activities that require added strength, but these are not sports the average person will engage in regularly over a lifetime.

Powerlifters can benefit from training for power, as well as strength, although this would be done mostly in the off-season. Many powerlifters do not regularly engage in other forms of training (for example, flexibility, aerobic conditioning), but a certain amount of this is helpful if for no other reason than to add the benefits for later in life, after the competitive career is over.

Power Sports

Weightlifting-specific training is popular with many athletes and coaches engaged in *power sports* (football, basketball, volleyball, track and field, weightlifting). It is here that the direct application of these types of lifts is most beneficial. While a baseball or basketball player does not need to focus on moving heavy objects, certain weightlifting training may be adapted to assist in the improvement of sport-specific skills that originate in the hips and core musculature.

Power-oriented sports require quick muscular action and adequate strength in order to produce power. All athletes involved in power sports need to address power development in their training in order to maximize potential. How best to go about this depends on a number of factors.

Quality practice of a power-oriented sport emphasizes power and maintaining a sharp, sport-specific execution. For example, actual volleyball practice aids the beginner in the development of a better vertical jump. Part of this improvement is related to neural adaptation or the training of the brain and the body to learn how to contract the muscles involved in jumping.

However, there is a limit to how much "natural" improvement can be expected. Much depends on where you start in terms of experience, your levels of strength, and your potential to get stronger. Some very important research coming out of the Cincinnati Sports Medicine and Orthopaedic Center confirms that young girls, in particular, run a risk of increased ACL (anterior cruciate ligament) injury from a lack of strength and stability. This "weak link" manifests itself particularly in jump landing. So, simply encouraging jumping without addressing quality controls and supplemental strengthening may actually lead to an injury.

Adding resistance training to sport-specific training on the field or court can be very beneficial to power-sport athletes. All other factors being equal, a power athlete who gets stronger even through general (nonspecific, nonpower) resistance training will probably outperform a player who simply practices the sport.

Most sport coaches and athletes today embrace the use of a generic resistance training program, if for no other reason than injury prevention. This may involve free weights, resistance training machines, or other forms of resistance. Repetitions tend toward 10 or 12, which is more than what sport science tells us will create absolute strength.

Many coaches who encourage general resistance training programs do not believe in the use of "explosive" or power-oriented movements in the weight room. This may be because of their lack of familiarity with the proper and safe ways to perform these lifts, their lack of proper equipment, or their philosophical opposition to this form of training. These coaches generally encourage a low number of sets per exercise, with a dependence on many seated or supported exercises using plate-loaded or weight stack machines. The repetitions are normally performed quite slowly, with an effort to produce muscular fatigue at about 12 repetitions.

In recent years the emphasis on very slow flexion and extension of a joint throughout its range of motion has received a lot of attention. Such slow training, while enjoying some fadlike acceptance at present, is not specific to any speed of movement you'll execute on the playing field or court. Although these slow protocols are certainly better than no resistance training at all, they ignore the commonly accepted practice of increasing speed strength in the gym.

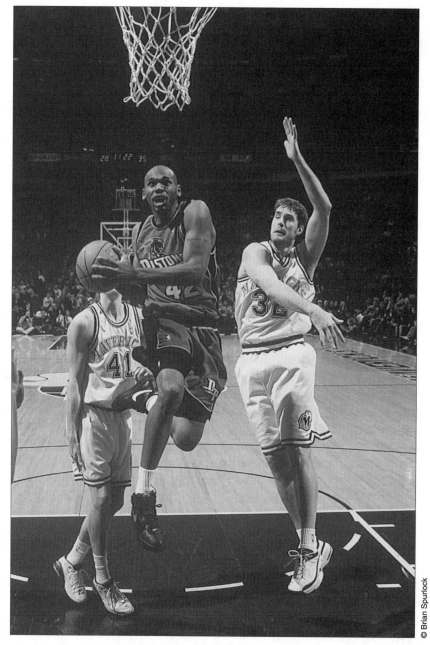

© Brian Spurlock

Explosive weightlifting gives you the edge over your opponent before you get on the court.

Power training in the weight room allows for the development of strength and power at the same time. With the addition to other power development exercises and sport-specific agility drills and practice, all your bases are covered.

The weightlifting movements highlighted in this book specifically train explosive muscular actions, particularly of the lower body. Performing the snatch, clean, or jerk in an explosive manner with appropriate resistance will train specifically the muscular actions clearly related to the production of vertical force.

True enough, most football players have little use for pure vertical force, although this varies by position. However, we can't practice the snatch or the clean in a horizontal position. Nevertheless, improving the ability to propel the body rapidly upward can improve the ability to propel the body forward, as in running or coming off the line. The joint (ankle, knee, hip) angles involved are similar as well.

Particularly tall basketball or volleyball players probably do not need to train the full range of motion required for these lifts, as jumps are executed from a lesser angle of flexion of the ankle, knee, and hip joints. Additionally, getting into position to lift a barbell from the floor can be quite difficult because of limb length and flexibility issues. In this case, performing snatch or clean movements with the bar off the floor (from blocks or the "hang" position) or simply performing partial movements (high pulls) will be sufficient to maintain an explosive, speed-strength movement more specific to basketball or volleyball.

Train for Power

The terms *speed strength* (force developed rapidly or at high velocities) and *explosive strength* (the ability to exert maximal forces in minimal time) have appeared in recent years. The use of these additional terms can make a discussion of power even more confusing. Just remember, the amount of power you generate depends on two factors: strength and speed. A very strong athlete lacking in FT fibers will not demonstrate outstanding power. Conversely, someone with a high percentage of FT fibers, but who is weak, will not display good power, especially against resistance.

The ability to generate great power quite often separates the winners from the also-rans in many sports. Two shot-putters may weigh the same and demonstrate equal strength in the weight room, yet perform quite differently in the ring. Or a smaller, lighter shot-putter may outperform the stronger, more heavily muscled competitor. The answer lies in how much power is produced. To maximize your athletic success, you must determine if your sport requires more skill, strength, power, or a combination of these factors. Then you need to spend your time training appropriately.

Some coaches discourage the use of "explosive" lifts, referencing concerns ranging from "football players don't play with a barbell on the field" to "explosive lifts are dangerous." Over the years I've found that one of the biggest hurdles to acceptance is the fact that many coaches simply do not have the skills necessary to safely and correctly teach these movements. And I will agree that having an athlete hurt in the weight room is unnecessary and undesirable.

Weightlifters are among the most powerful athletes around. While many of you do not plan to take up weightlifting as your primary sport, you can safely use weightlifting-specific movements in your training program to great effect. Keep in mind, though, that this type of training requires the same attention to detail as your primary sport, even though it is only an adjunct part of your overall training program.

All good weightlifters did not come to the platform on day 1 with the power characteristics necessary to succeed. They train specifically for power through the use of snatch, clean, jerk, and related lifts, all of which have a positive effect on power production. In addition, while training with these lifts, they get stronger, and so can you. To get both stronger and more powerful in the gym provides the most time-efficient manner of training, compared to training these qualities separately.

I'll address *plyometric* training in the next chapter. Plyometric training has a positive effect on both strength and speed. And since the classic weightlifting movements are actually plyometric movements with heavier resistance, you gain multiple benefits in your quest for added power. Weightlifting is not the only way to train, but it is an important part of the equation.

Combining Weightlifting and Plyometrics

Power is the one ingredient that often spells success in many sports. We've talked about the variables involved in power production. You've heard convincing arguments that the best way to resistance train for a power-oriented sport is with sport-specific power movements, along with practicing your chosen sport.

Simply following strength/power athlete training programs is not always the complete answer. A boxer or baseball player, for example, may benefit from performing explosive weightlifting-specific exercises; however, neither athlete is going to perform in any way resembling a weightlifter. While they could get better at snatch and clean-and-jerk movements, the amount of transfer to their sport may be less than, say, that of a volleyball or basketball player. Thus, boxers or baseball players would need to include other exercises more specific to their activities.

Sport coaches and sport scientists always look for new, better, or different ways to improve performance by training power and sport-specific movements. What is now popularly known as *plyometrics* was discovered and refined over the past 25 or so years. This form of training offers some positive additions to athletes seeking improvement in power.

Fancy Word, Simple Concept

From the Greek words *plio* (more) and *metric* (to measure), we see that plyometric literally means "to increase measurement." In theory, plyometric training enables a muscle or muscle group to reach its maximum force in the shortest period of time. This certainly has direct application to sport.

For an activity to be plyometric, it must include what is known as a *stretch-shortening cycle (SSC)*. This refers to the process of loading a muscle eccentrically (the muscle lengthens against tension), followed rapidly by a concentric muscle action (the muscle shortens against resistance). The initial rapid eccentric motion allows the subsequent concentric action to exceed that which it could produce alone.

Let's look at a couple of examples of plyometric effects. At the midstride point in running you are momentarily suspended in air. Your shoe comes in contact with the running surface, followed by a flexion of your hip, knee, and ankle joints. This flexion helps to absorb the shock forces that are many times greater than your own body weight. This absorption phase includes a slight lowering of your body as the muscles act as a shock absorber. This causes an eccentric muscle action in the muscles of your lower body that arrests the downward motion by "applying the brakes." Without this eccentric braking action, your body would collapse to the ground.

Momentum and other muscles (hamstrings, gluteals) of your front leg carry your body forward over your planted foot. As your body passes over your foot, your former forward leg now becomes your rear leg and it propels your body forward by pushing against the running surface. This pushing is accomplished by a concentric muscle action of those hip and leg muscles that had previously been stretched eccentrically.

Another example of the plyometric effect is the standard vertical jump test described in chapter 2. This test normally involves what is called a countermovement (that is, the lowering of the body before the upward jump by flexing the ankles, knees, and hips). This countermovement produces a stretch-shortening cycle, with the joints flexed and the body lowered several inches (a fairly natural movement for anyone planning to jump). This cycle causes the quadriceps muscles in the front of the thighs to stretch, along with various muscles of the lower leg.

The time required for the athlete to "brake" the downward motion and reverse the force to push against the floor is called the *amortization phase*. The shorter this turnaround phase, the quicker the direction is changed, and the better the vertical jump result. The slower the amortization phase, the less likely the subject is to gain any benefit from the initial lowering of the body.

The eccentric action and the amortization phase are crucial to the success of any plyometric action. During this phase, the body's natural defense against excessive stretching, called the *stretch reflex,* kicks in. This is an involuntary response that protects the body from going beyond its safe and natural limits. Once the muscles have stretched as far as they can go, the stretch reflex causes them to tighten again.

The stretch reflex kicks in upon detecting a rapid initiation of the stretch, thus limiting the amount of stretch. But since muscle is elastic, this stretching (much like a rubber band) stores elastic energy that can be released when, and if, the muscle contracts quickly after the stretch. If the contraction does not follow quickly after the stretch, the energy is dissipated. Because of the elastic quality of muscle tissue, the eccentric action followed quickly by a concentric action increases the contractile force of muscles beyond what would occur if the movement were performed without the stretch-shortening portion.

Identifying this phenomenon, coaches and sport scientists began to exploit this type of training. Jumps of various types became part of the training programs for athletes involved in lower-body performance (such as soccer, cycling, sprinting). Coaches of athletes more dependent on upper-body speed and quickness (boxers, shot-putters, tennis players) created exercises to plyometrically train the muscles of the arms, chest, shoulders, and torso. This could include performing push-ups with a clap between reps or, while lying supine, catching a weighted medicine ball dropped from several feet overhead and then quickly throwing it back up.

Comparing Plyometric and Explosive Weight Training

Both external resistance and plyometric training help strengthen the body's muscles. Plyometric training includes a *ballistic* component not available in many resistance exercises. Ballistic refers to launching an object (medicine ball, barbell, body weight) explosively into space. This can provide some advantages over traditional barbell or dumbbell exercises. However, launching free weights presents a risk to equipment, facilities, or others, to say nothing of being rather unpopular with gym owners and their lawyers.

Let's say a shot-putter or boxer wanted to develop more explosive power in extending his arms to the front. Traditionally we'd look to a bench press or incline press for the strengthening component. Performed quickly (with a lighter resistance), the implement (barbell or dumbbells) could accelerate quickly, but you have to begin to slow down the extension before reaching the end of the range of motion. Otherwise, you risk injury to the shoulders and elbows. Since the bench press is such a short range of motion, you may spend more time slowing down the lift than accelerating it.

Throwing a medicine ball from either a flat bench or an incline bench allows you to create the force necessary to hurl the ball a pretty good distance. Obviously, if you're lying supine on a flat bench, someone needs to

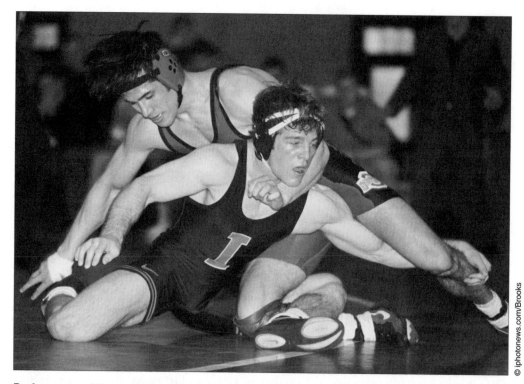

Performance of the explosive lifts closely resembles the moves necessary to compete on the wrestling mat.

catch the medicine ball or it will return to hit you. This ballistic training is considered sport specific and power oriented, creating a much more appropriate exercise than simply the bench press. However, a blend of both types of training seems to be best.

A wrestler can perform power snatches or power cleans or any type of related pulling exercise. This will train the lower body and simulate the muscular and joint action needed to pick up and move an opponent. Similar training is performed with wrestling "dummies" in the workout room. The barbell provides more appropriate progressive resistance; the dummy provides a more realistic object to move. The barbell cannot be safely thrown; the dummy can.

So, which form of training is used really depends on the phase of training you are in and how that relates to variety in a periodized training program. As we'll learn later, variety, especially for advanced athletes, is critical to continued improvement.

Plyometric Exercises

As you'll see when we closely examine the technique of weightlifting movements, any properly performed snatch, clean, or jerk produces a plyometric effect for the lower body. In fact, modifications in the pulling technique over the past 40 years exploit this plyometric advantage. During either the pulling phase of the snatch or clean or in the forceful execution of the jerk, the lifter must quickly lower the body, "hit the brakes," and then powerfully push the body and the barbell in the opposite direction. Remember the notion of "jumping with the barbell in the hands."

As an overall category of exercises, plyometric training includes weightlifting. Nonweightlifting plyometric training must include some form of external resistance (a medicine ball or body weight are the most likely objects) to provide resistance. External resistance objects used in plyometric exercise are somewhat limited in size and weight, whereas a barbell can be continually adjusted to a heavier resistance.

Many athletes and coaches think only of jumping exercises when they discuss plyometric training. And, sure enough, most jump training is plyometric in effect. This may include single jumps or bounds (repeated jump efforts), jumps onto or over an object, side-to-side jumping, or single-leg or double-leg takeoffs or landings. Literally dozens of plyometric exercises are available for any muscle group. As you can see, this type of training can be easily customized to a particular sport.

When plyometric training is mentioned, many coaches and athletes think only of the most advanced form, called *depth jumps*. This requires you to step off an elevated box or bench (optimally from .5 to 1.0 meter in height), land solidly on both feet, and then jump upward or outward. The additional shock effect of jumping from such a height is considered the most advanced form of plyometric training and should not be engaged in by novices.

The scientific literature frequently mentions a recommendation that individuals be able to squat 1.5 times their body weight before engaging in plyometric training. In the case of young athletes, this is an extremely high amount of strength to demonstrate before encouraging jump training. Youngsters regularly engage in daily plyometric activities (jump rope, running), yet none of them would be expected to squat this much weight. This book introduces explosive lifting movements that are plyometric in nature long before the ability to squat such a heavy weight is gained. The need to squat 1.5 times one's body weight is probably a more appropriate suggestion before attempting depth jumps, especially from heights greater than half a meter. This kind of strength demonstrates that the muscles and connective tissue are strong enough to handle a higher level of intensity.

The Cincinnati Sports Medicine and Orthopaedic Center has focused on plyometric and explosive resistance training to strengthen young muscles and connective tissue. This is especially useful when working with young athletes lacking adequate strength or proper mechanics to allow them to jump and land properly. Careful use of progressive plyometric exercise, including a longer "stick" position when landing, allows for isometric muscle action to strengthen the muscles at that joint angle where the young athlete may be weakest.

Weightlifting or Plyometrics?

Athletes and coaches often ask the question Which type of training is better? Both weightlifting training and pure plyometric training share a number of similarities. There is room for both activities in a power athlete's training program, but the percentage of each type of training will depend on the sport involved and the time of the year. For many sports a combination of weightlifting exercises, plyometric drills, and both specific and nonspecific (remedial) resistance training methods may work best.

Weightlifters

Weightlifters have traditionally jumped and sprinted as part of their general physical training regimen, often more heavily in the off-season. It is not unusual for lifters to perform some jumping several days per week during any phase, either before or after weightlifting training. When I coached the USA weightlifting team at the Olympic Training Center in Colorado Springs, we met on the track at 8:00 A.M. for some general training. This included a good deal of jumping, flexibility, and general mobility exercises. Being up and active at this hour assured a more positive workout environment at the 11:00 A.M. training session. Often the lifters would engage in a few more minutes of plyometric training at the end of the 4:00–6:00 P.M. workout.

Most lifters constantly monitor the overall state of their knees. So much training for the snatch and clean-and-jerk, along with daily bouts of squatting, can leave the knees sensitive to additional stresses. We monitored jump training carefully and backed off much of this activity, either in terms of volume (foot contacts per workout) or intensity (effort in the concentric jump phase) depending on the lifter's overall "knee health." We did not encourage depth jumps unless the lifter's knees were totally pain-free.

Many successful weightlifters include some jumping drills in their daily or weekly training programs. Simple single- or double-leg jumps or bounds are used, as are jumps onto or over an object or a series of objects. Single-leg versions are particularly helpful for athletes who display asymmetrical leg strength.

Movements such as catching a medicine ball between the legs and then rapidly throwing it overhead with both the lower body and lower back benefit the trunk extensors. Exercises for either the trunk extensors or flexors must be carefully supervised, as a large range of motion will negate much of the plyometric effect. The range of motion for the eccentric portion of these exercises must be kept short.

Because weightlifting success is largely due to lower-body strength and power, the typical lifter does not normally focus on upper-body plyometrics.

Other Athletes

Because many power athletes from track and field depend on both lower- and upper-body strength and speed, combining weightlifting and plyometrics is wise. Additional attention to rotational power is a must.

The needs of football players are clearly defined by their position. For instance, linemen (both defensive and offensive) need to fend off opposing players with their upper bodies. Receivers and backs will have more focus on starting speed, change of direction, and occasional vertical requirements. Quarterbacks are concerned with improvement of their throwing arm, kickers, with the dominant leg.

So, you can see that plyometric training is important for power-based athletes. And, as we've discussed, this same group can benefit from explosive weightlifting training.

Careful Blend of Both Methods

Plyometric training provides an excellent stimulus for increased power. Additionally, this type of training can be fun and is a nice diversion from the sometimes routine workouts in a weight room. However, you'll probably find it best to devote more or less time to plyometrics depending on your sport and its specific requirements.

Generally, physical training progresses from general to specific. This means that the further away from a season or peak performance you are, the more general training will occur. In a power-oriented sport, you want to reach your peak power performance in-season and close to the competition that means the most to you. A cyclist peaking for the national championships in the summer does not need to be at her best in December or January, traditionally part of the off-season.

It is normally recommended that you first prepare the muscles through general training, which consists of a high to moderate volume of work at moderate intensity. As intensity of effort increases, you should back off a bit on volume. Trying to increase intensity while volume is high is courting injury. So, plyometric training, which is normally considered to be high intensity (otherwise it is not truly plyometric), takes a back seat in the off-season. It comes to the forefront as the season approaches and is an integral part of the in-season phase of training.

How Important Is Plyometric Training?

Like resistance training in general and explosive resistance training in particular, plyometric training is another controversial topic that divides coaches and sport scientists. Despite a large volume of scientific work that endorses plyometric training for power-oriented athletes, some people, for whatever reason, attempt to downplay this training's effectiveness.

Like knowing how to snatch or clean-and-jerk, I look to plyometric training as another ingredient in my coaching recipe book. I probably would not focus an undue amount of time on this method of training unless I worked with an athlete who could benefit from it. I agree with many that this is a very intense form of exercise, particularly when using something like depth jumps, and it should be used appropriately. On the other hand, I recognize the benefits of offering a different means of training to athletes, and I know that jump training can help an athlete unfamiliar with power production.

A few years ago I had the opportunity to work with one of the outstanding women cyclists in the United States. Being a former triathlete, she excelled at long-distance events but suffered in group sprints. Unfortunately, much of women's racing in this country involves the pack staying together until near the end of the race, then field-sprinting to the line.

We had worked a season or two on getting stronger, primarily in the lower body. But, because of her long in-season and a failure to maintain resistance training except in the off-season, this rider received minimal benefits from short-term squatting. So, at the end of her workouts at least twice a week we began some simple jump training on the stairs leading out of the Olympic Training Center weight room.

Typical of one who has little jumping experience, the rider had a certain psychological block toward the activity. She appeared overwhelmed by the task of jumping up the stairs two at a time. Patience prevailed, and she soon conquered this challenge. We then moved to jumping three and finally four steps at a time or doing bounds of two or three steps to the top of two flights of stairs. After the more serious weight training was over, this was the prescribed manner for exiting the gym. Eventually it became a relaxed and fun 15 minutes of additional training.

In the final season in which I was involved in her training, the rider went off to the national team early season races. She reported that now when the group came to the sprint, she felt she had not only more physical tools to compete but also the mind-set of what an explosive exercise felt like. Her results improved drastically, although she never became either a great sprinter or an accomplished stair-jumper. As discussed in chapter 2, she did not increase the number of fast-twitch fibers she had, but she sure learned how to use those that were available.

Knowing what the stretch-shortening cycle feels like and knowing how to apply maximum power after an eccentric contraction is a positive trait for many athletes. Plyometric training can facilitate that awareness and contribute to better performance. So, while you should not get carried away and perform an excessive amount of plyometric training, the sensible integration of this training modality into the overall plan makes a lot of sense.

We have now covered the issues of strength, power, and speed strength. You're now ready to discover the main premise of this book, the use of explosive weightlifting training for improved performance.

Building a Technique Base

Success in weightlifting depends on two criteria: the establishment of excellent technique and significant gains in strength and power. Some detractors of weightlifting say top performance in this sport is all technique, which is simply not true. Many technique differences and mistakes occur even at the highest level of competition.

Your first step in learning weightlifting movements must be the development of optimal technique. It is much easier to gain strength and power after you've learned how to perform the lifts. The time to learn many of the intricacies of the snatch and clean-and-jerk is in the early teen years. Many older athletes with outstanding strength and power have found the mastery of weightlifting technique frustrating.

Coaches and sport scientists in various countries have examined closely the best sequence for young athletes learning weightlifting technique. Some have argued for learning the snatch first, some the clean, some the jerk; yet others have suggested first learning assistance exercises. There are pluses and minuses to all of these approaches, but no method is clearly superior to another. For our purposes, I'll introduce the lifts in the order they are contested.

Learning theory tells us that the human mind and body learn a new skill several ways. These include:

1. *The Whole Method.* The entire movement is taught as a single unit, without breaking down a complex motion into simpler segments. An example is swinging a baseball bat. There is no reason to teach the swing in phases, as it is impossible to pick up the motion from a partially executed swing. Teaching a more complex motion with this method, however, presents many problems, as a newcomer cannot be expected to master a complicated action easily. This then leads to the reinforcement of numerous errors that are difficult to eliminate over time.

2. *The Part Method.* Some complex actions are easily taught by breaking them down into several, more easily learned segments. Complex, multiple-joint movements often can be taught one stage at a time, paying particular attention to mastering the more complex parts first, then building together the entire movement, and ending with the simpler parts. While many coaches try to teach explosive lifts in this manner, the result is often a series of segmented portions that lack one coordinated execution. Performing these lifts in segments is very frustrating and inefficient for the novice.

3. *The Whole-Part-Whole Method.* This method allows for the initial imitation of the entire motion, followed by concentrated practice of segmented portions of a movement, then finally putting the entire movement back together. I prefer this method as it allows a new lifter to initially experience the entire lift (with only light weights), but then learn the finer points of proper technique before bad habits become ingrained. After mastering the most difficult portions in isolation, the full movement is fluid and well-coordinated.

Importance of Proper Technique

Early weightlifting competitions consisted of five lifts (the press, snatch, clean-and-jerk, one-hand snatch, and one-hand clean-and-jerk). This was quickly trimmed to three lifts by eliminating the one-hand lifts. The press (eliminated by 1973) and the clean-and-jerk were largely strength-oriented lifts, the snatch being more technically demanding. The snatch was often a relatively ignored component of training, with lifters spending most of their training time getting stronger. Early weightlifting champions displayed outstanding strength and speed, but their actual lifting technique often left much to be desired. As international competition grew, technique became a much more important consideration. Gone were the early champions who simply hauled the bar off the platform with little finesse. Today's winning lifters are much more fluid in their movements.

The snatch and clean-and-jerk are multiple-joint, total-body movements that include both pulling and pushing on the barbell. Because some parts of the lifts are more complex than others and some parts require more speed of movement, it makes sense to break the lifts into segments, learning the most difficult parts first. Several successful weightlifting countries, most notably the former Soviet Union, consider this the best way to learn the lifts. USA Weightlifting uses a segmental means of teaching the lifts to coaches and athletes.

Regardless of the approach used, all initial efforts to imitate the snatch and clean-and-jerk lifts should be practiced only with a broom stick or dowel, gradually moving to an empty weightlifting bar. A beginner does not need the distraction of an actual barbell while learning.

As a new lifter, you need to realize that these lifts are rapid, fluid motions and not choppy, segmented pieces loosely linked together. You must focus on the end result—getting the bar overhead or on your shoulders in a fast, powerful manner. Many well-intentioned but poorly trained coaches have taught the lifts in a jerky, automated fashion reminiscent of the old notion that the snatch and clean consist of a "first" pull, a "second" pull, and a "third" pull. Although the pull does goes through several stages, this way of teaching can severely hinder progress, making the movement choppy. In reality the pulling motion for the snatch and the clean should be viewed as a fast, explosive action similar to starting a sprint out of the blocks. True, the pull becomes faster and faster as the bar rises from the floor, but this is not done in segments. To start deliberately slowly and try to build speed may keep a lifter from creating enough power to maximize performance. The ability to start powerfully and finish explosively is the key to success, although this skill takes time to learn and will vary with individual abilities and size.

As a newcomer to this type of lifting, you can gain an appreciation of the lifts by seeing them performed by experienced lifters. Check with USA Weightlifting, the governing body for the sport of weightlifting in the United States, for a member club or competitive opportunities near you. If you can't get to a live demonstration of the sport, look for a videotaped or filmed depiction of the lifts. Study the sequential photographs in this book to learn what happens at each stage within the lifts.

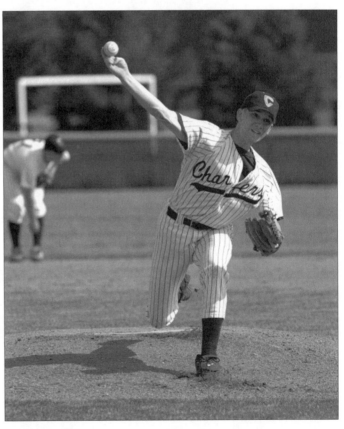

Learn the snatch and clean-and-jerk lifts as a comprehensive, explosive movement and translate the benefits to your sport.

And, simply reading the technical instructions (chapters 5, 6, and 7) and following the learning process I've outlined in this book will have you doing both lifts in a very short period of time. Just keep in mind as you look at still pictures that, properly done, these lifts are performed with nearly blinding speed.

Ideally an athlete who wants to learn the snatch and clean-and-jerk lifts should enlist the help of a properly qualified weightlifting coach. You can learn a lot by simply watching, but it is crucial to watch the lifts performed correctly *and* have the lifting process explained properly. This can present a challenge, even when a coach claims to understand weightlifting technique and may have a credential to indicate he has taken part in a coaching certification program. Successful modeling at this early stage can be the single key to success in learning these complicated skills.

Evolution of Pulling Technique

As weightlifting has evolved from a fairly brute strength sport to one of combined explosive power and strength, the method used to elevate heavier weights has gone through many changes. You can still perform a snatch or clean-and-jerk by simply picking the barbell up off the floor with little concern for technique, but you won't get very far. Moreover, you certainly won't gain the benefits of doing the lifts explosively and correctly.

Toward a More Efficient Technique

Since weightlifting involves two pulling movements, a good deal of the training time is devoted to pulling the barbell from the floor to overhead (snatch), to the chest (clean), or somewhere along the torso (partial pulling exercises). However, the mere act of correctly picking up the bar is more complex than it may appear initially. How the bar is lifted is crucial to mastering proper technique and maintaining progress.

Biomechanists have studied for many years the style of pulling used in weightlifting. A fairly unified body of knowledge exists in terms of the most efficient lifting style. Of course, there is plenty of room for individual differences, as well. Depending on one's own body size and limb proportions, coaching style, or in some cases cultural effects, two successful snatches may arrive at the same basic end position through much different means.

Early technical rules forbid lifters from touching any part of the body with the bar before its arrival at the final position. This "clean" motion is how the clean-and-jerk got its name. This was done to differentiate between the clean-and-jerk and an unofficial lift, the *continental*-and-jerk. The latter lift involved first pulling the bar to the belt, then using a combined effort of the legs and upper body to pull the bar from the belt to the shoulders.

The S-Pull

With records going higher each year, sport scientists determined that successful lifts showed a barbell trajectory that did not follow a perfectly straight line, although that is obviously the shortest distance between two points. It was determined that the most successful performances reflected a trajectory that looked something like an elongated letter *S*. Don't get confused here: The bar is not actively swung in or out, as this can quickly lead to failure. It is much easier to manipulate the body, which normally weighs less, around the bar than vice versa.

The first (liftoff) part of the S-pull results in a slight inward sweep of the bar toward the shins, sometimes resulting in contact of the lower leg (shin) by the bar. Prior to about 1960 judges were required to refuse such a technical rule violation. Later, seeing the common nature of this trait and realizing it did not assist an athlete to lift more weight, the technical rules were modified to allow the lifter to contact the shins during the pull without penalty. Any contact of the body above the knee by the barbell remained illegal.

After the initial liftoff, with the bar at about knee height and the knees nearly straight, this early style resulted in the barbell rising fairly straight as the shoulders and torso were elevated by hip extension. Such a motion ignores the strong quadriceps muscles of the thighs and often results in premature use of the even weaker arm muscles. To lift progressively heavier weights, an important subtle change slowly crept into weightlifting technique.

Previously, the hips remained far from the bar. To lift heavier weights it was clear that the hips needed to drive inward and upward. While driving the hips in this fashion made sense biomechanically, depending on the lifter's body proportions, this motion brought the hips and thighs dangerously close to, or in contact with, the bar. Contact between the body and the bar remained against the technical rules of the day.

Such contact was particularly evident in the rapidly rising performances of the lifters from Japan. Often exhibiting a relatively long torso with short arms and legs, the Japanese produced excellent results in the snatch and clean by making several technical modifications. The Japanese began what became known as the "frog style" of pulling, which consisted of placing the heels together, turning the toes and knees out a considerable amount, lowering the hips quite close to the heels, and then beginning the pull. This posture counteracted the otherwise negative effect of a long torso. By adopting this posture, the Japanese lifters kept the torso much straighter in the pull, so they could effectively snatch or clean using their dominant strong levers, the legs.

One side effect of this style was a brushing of the barbell against the upper thighs as the hips came toward the bar. With the arms straight, the torso nearly vertical, and the ankles, knees, and hips slightly flexed, the lifter is in the strongest possible position to jump violently upward with the barbell. This is a much stronger position than simply trying to extend the hip through a wide range of motion followed by pulling with the arms.

Largely through the scientific efforts of Dave Webster, the Scottish national weightlifting coach, the weightlifting world became aware of this new evolution in pulling technique. Webster measured and wrote extensively on how certain lifters brought their hips to the bar, thus resulting in a stronger biomechanical position to exert force. He was quick to point out, however, that if this technique resulted in contact between the bar and the thighs, this was a violation of the rules.

Initially, the technical officials either did not see what was happening or chose not to enforce the rules. Rather quickly weightlifters from many nations adopted this technique, although the "frog style" starting position was not used successfully by many since the nuances were not fully understood or appropriate for every build. Unfortunately, numerous "expert" coaches claimed that lifters were now simply bouncing the bar off their thighs and this became the rage. Such advice set the sport of weightlifting back technically for many years, especially in the United States. Bouncing the bar off the thighs causes a deflection in the bar's trajectory, creating a misdirected snatch or clean. Such a deflection also slows the overall lift.

As with contact below the knees, the technical rules were eventually modified to allow a brush of the thighs by the bar but not "violent contact." Later, as this technique continued to be modified, contact with the "lap," or lower abdomen was allowed, initially for the snatch, now for both lifts.

Once the lifter explosively extends the ankles, knees, and hips, the bar proceeds close to the torso in a nearly vertical line. At the same time, the lifter is pulling under the rising barbell. The barbell loops over at the top of the snatch or clean and returns to approximately the same location, in terms of horizontal displacement, as its starting point. The "hook," or top portion of the S-pull, is more pronounced in the snatch, where the barbell is located behind the head. In the clean, the hook merely places the bar on the shoulders.

Variations in Barbell Trajectory

As mentioned earlier, there is a great deal of variation in how even champion weightlifters lift the barbell. Most athletes who use explosive lifting for improvement in their sport should strive for traditional weightlifting technique. You don't need to try the latest theory in weightlifting-specific technique; just do the lifts in a manner that allows you to safely and effectively get stronger and more powerful.

In terms of lifting the bar overhead or to the chest, figure 4.1a is what the traditional barbell trajectory looks like. Emulation of this pathway will lead to improved performance in the snatch and clean lifts.

In recent years some weightlifting coaches have unfortunately advocated what they call a "jump back" style. In this case, the lifter's shoulders finish the pull behind the bar, resulting in a jump back to catch the weight, which

FIGURE 4.1 a-c   The S-shaped pull, rearward trajectory, and forward displacement.

has been directed rearward (figure 4.1b). While some very good lifters choose to jump backward, whether this is an optimal effect remains to be determined. The typical athlete looking to simply learn explosive lifts for improved sport performance need not copy this trajectory.

Some lifters jump forward to catch a bar that is swung or drifts too far in front of the body (figure 4.1c). There is near universal agreement that jumping forward is not an efficient way to lift. If the lifter consistently jumps forward under a snatch or clean to catch the barbell, some basic mistake in the liftoff phase or in the scooping action that follows needs to be corrected. Often this is related to an improper starting position.

"Double Knee Bend" Debate

As we've just discussed, a technically proficient modern weightlifter manipulates his or her body into a more favorable biomechanical position to elevate greater weights than could otherwise be lifted. It's much easier to move the body around than to try to redirect the bar's path.

It's important to repeat the traits of the S-pull technique. All lifters begin the snatch or clean with the ankles, knees, and hips flexed (bent). In the initial liftoff stage the barbell separates from the floor and arrives at the knees through extension (straightening) of these three joints.

From here the bar is elevated by extending the hips. To get into a powerful jumping position, the ankles, knees, and hips are again bent (flexed). In the early 1970s this became known simply as the "double knee bend" method of lifting. It might just as easily have been called the "double ankle bend" or "double hip bend" style of lifting.

Early on, lifters were encouraged to initially place the bar on the lower third of the thigh. The idea was to then slide the bar into a position higher on the thighs as the body moved into a more effective jumping position. The location of initial bar contact on the thighs was different for the snatch and the clean because of the variation in grip width. Such a dragging motion slowed the bar speed considerably. And, any slowing of the bar's elevation restricts the amount of weight snatched or cleaned.

Lifters and coaches then went to work to correct this problem with the use of oil, water, talc, or other lubricants on the thighs. This presented even further problems that resulted in more technical rules that forbade the use of such substances.

The most advanced weightlifting countries further modified technique so that the bar, for the most part, avoids any dragging on the thighs, yet still may make contact even up to the lower abdominal (lap) area. In this case, the body arrives in an efficient jumping position without slowing down the bar, yet the hips are still used to impart a powerful upward thrust to the bar.

This thrusting action, not the contact of the bar on the thighs or lower abdomen, results in a noticeable auditory cue for insightful coaches and athletes. Especially in training, where experienced lifters may not use collars to secure weights on the end of the bar, this ringing sound is noticeable at the same time the lower extremities execute a violent upward thrust. Unfortunately, many people confuse this sound with "banging the bar" and deflecting the upward motion needed to succeed with a heavy lift.

Experts agree that the ankles, knees, and hips must bend or rebend for the lifter to arrive at an effective jumping position. Some claim, however, this action cannot be taught; it simply occurs naturally in some athletes. They contend it is merely a reaction of the stretch reflex phenomenon in the hamstrings when the bar is at knee height, the knees are nearly straight, and the shoulders are in front of the bar.

The stretch reflex that occurs in this position does facilitate the rebending of the lower body prior to explosively jumping upward. Beginners, however, are unlikely to automatically demonstrate this action while learning technique. Novices repeatedly drill technique with very light resistances, and it is very rare to witness a beginner place the bar anywhere close to the thighs. It is much more tempting to use the hip extensors and even the arms to elevate light weights. If the beginner does not learn this movement early on, it's unlikely it will simply occur properly when he lifts near maximum weights after several months of training.

Those lifters who successfully transitioned from an era when thigh contact was prohibited to the modern-day pulling style demonstrated that this skill could be learned. I think the technique, which is not much different from the countermovement experienced in a vertical jump, can be taught and successfully learned. You'll have the experience of learning this technique in the next chapters, long before you attempt to lift a heavy weight.

Basic Pulling Technique

Pulling the barbell either overhead in the snatch or to the chest in the clean requires a coordinated series of sequential stages to occur correctly. When you see an elite lifter snatch or clean-and-jerk a record weight, often it looks very easy and less than a true maximum effort. However, a small error at any stage in the pulling process will often result in a failed effort. For this reason you should be sure to study carefully all the details and strive to learn the pulling technique properly.

Starting Position

The human body is not designed to effectively pull a heavy weight from the floor to overhead (snatch) or to the chest (clean). If it were only a matter of lifting the bar from the floor and standing up with it, as in the deadlift (a competitive lift in the sport of powerlifting), technique would be simple. In the deadlift, powerlifters wear footwear with no heel, stand with their shins right against the bar, and keep their balance toward the heels. They want to keep the torso as erect as possible, thus using the hips and thighs to pick the weight up. If a weightlifter were to start like this, she would invariably have trouble fixing the barbell overhead or on the chest, due mostly to an inability to jump vertically while positioned on the heels.

We now know that the best weightlifters do not lift the bar straight from the floor. With room for individual differences, it is generally suggested that you place your feet about hip-width apart and align the bar over the metatarsal phalangeal joint (MTP) before squatting down to place your hands on the bar (figure 4.2). Once you grasp the bar in this position, you'll feel some awkwardness in being able to lift a heavy weight from this posture. But, this is the place to start.

Many beginners, particularly those without top-quality coaches, fail to learn how to lift efficiently from this position. Novice lifters often "crowd the bar," more like a power-lifter, and may actually have the bar roll forward as they squat down into a starting position. It is much better to place the feet correctly and not have the bar roll as the starting position is taken. Awkward or not, remember that the bar is *not* going to be lifted straight up.

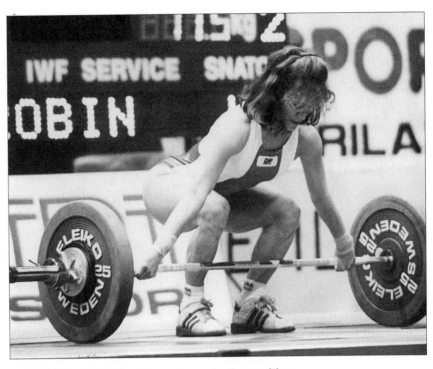

FIGURE 4.2   Robin Goad in a strong starting position.

Liftoff

The first part of the pull causes the barbell to come toward your shins a few centimeters. This is *not* an attempt to roll the bar or deliberately cause it to move backward. However, with your elbows directly over the barbell, your latissimus dorsi muscles contracted, and your scapulae retracted, the bar will arc backward toward the center line it naturally seeks as the liftoff occurs. The only joint movement during liftoff is a combined hip and knee extension. The concept of "pushing the platform away," while physically impossible, tends to keep your body in the proper position, with your shoulders and hips rising at the same pace.

Once the bar is back in a position that allows fairly straight upward movement, your hips and knees continue to extend and your shoulders are placed at their farthest position in front of the barbell, with the barbell approximately at knee height (figure 4.3). To get to this stage, your balance shifts slightly toward the center or rear part of your foot (not your heels), as opposed to the front part of your foot in the starting position.

Recently some lifters have utilized what I call a bow-legged style of pulling. This is not truly a frog style as the heels are not touching. The toes and knees point sharply outward, which allows for a fairly upright liftoff portion of the snatch or clean. Unlike either the frog style or conventional pulling technique, when the bar arrives at the knee level in this bow-legged style the lifter's shoulders are more directly over the bar instead of in front of the bar.

Scoop

Since the knees and ankles are nearly fully extended, the next part of the body to now contribute to the pull is the torso, which via hip extension

FIGURE 4.3   Hip and knee extension for liftoff.

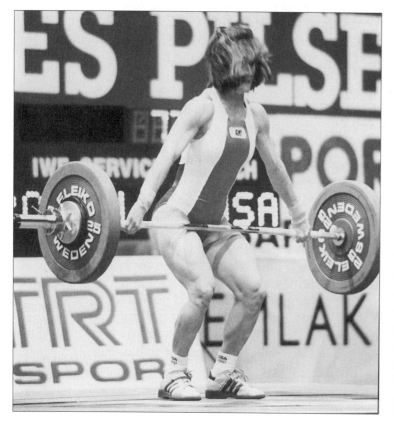

FIGURE 4.4   The "power position" is achieved by bending the ankles, knees, and hips.

extends to a fairly upright position. The posture with the bar at the knees places a great deal of stretch on the hamstring muscle group of the rear thigh. As your hips extend, a dorsiflexion of your ankles and flexion of the knee and hip joints occur, placing your knees under the barbell so that your balance returns to the front part of your foot (but not your toes). (See figure 4.4.) Be sure to keep your feet flat on the platform as long as possible. Premature elevation of the heels leads to an inefficient pulling motion.

The scoop is accomplished while still lifting the barbell in a motion mostly straight up. Keep the barbell clear of your thighs until your hips are placed well under the bar. This is a tremendously difficult maneuver to master and makes a properly performed snatch or clean an amazingly coordinated athletic feat to witness.

Due to the different posture when the bar is at knee height, the bow-legged style does not elicit the stretch reflex in the hamstrings. This eliminates the need to shift the body around the bar, but the barbell ends up in the same power, or jump, position.

Jump Phase

With your balance back toward the front part of your foot (but not on your toes), the barbell contacts your upper thigh or lower abdomen (in the snatch) or your mid- to upper thigh (in the clean). Your shoulders remain over the bar as long as possible. This is the "power position" and is very similar to a vertical jump motion while holding a barbell in your hands. A tremendous amount of power is created here, which is how the bar is elevated. (See figure 4.5.)

Now you perform a maximum-effort, explosive vertical jump, resulting in a triple extension of your ankle, knee, and hip joints. During this part of the lift the bar passes slightly in front of the vertical line created when the barbell was on the floor. The violent upward movement is accomplished with your lower body. Your arms remain straight as the trapezius muscles of your upper back quickly contract.

Pull-Under

Rather than deliberately attempting to pull the bar any higher with your arms (some of the weakest muscles in the body), you now accelerate your body weight *down against the rising bar*. This maneuver, which is actually very difficult to accomplish, can only be performed with your feet on the floor (figure 4.6). The reason for pulling under is simple: The bar will soon run out of momentum and you are in a very weak position to exert additional force to raise the bar. In the case of an experienced lifter, the barbell weighs more than the athlete, so it is much easier to pull the lighter weight of the body down against the heavier barbell.

In the past few years some coaches have emphasized jumping off the platform at this stage of the lift. They encourage lifters to stomp the feet or make a noticeable sound when landing on the platform. Many lifters, in an attempt to satisfy this request, sharply bend their hip and knee joints to draw the feet off the platform.

Think for a moment of a car leaving the highway under great speed and becoming airborne. Despite the driver's best efforts, no amount of pressure on the gas or brake pedals has any influence on the car; it simply becomes a missile. If your feet are off the ground while doing a snatch or clean, you cannot accelerate the downward pulling motion

FIGURE 4.5 Triple extension of the ankles, knees, and hips for a powerful jump.

FIGURE 4.6 A strong pull-under accelerates the body downward against the rising bar.

FIGURE 4.7   A solid catch requires strength and balance.

FIGURE 4.8   Recovery to a standing position.

of the body. Instead, you are in a free fall posture and will contact the floor in a semi-squat position, rather than actively pulling under.

A noticeable difference between top lifters and those in the lower ranks is the speed and efficiency with which the elite get under the bar. In chapters 5 and 6 I encourage you to learn the lifts without lifting your feet off the platform. After you learn the concept of pulling yourself under the bar, you may choose to experiment with a slight repositioning of the feet from the liftoff to the catch or rack of the bar. This depends on your own preferences and flexibility in the starting and receiving positions. Just remember, you can't pull against the bar when your feet are off the platform.

Catch

Pulling your body under the bar rapidly brings you into position under the barbell. Most weightlifters reposition their feet to achieve a comfortable squat position. The split style snatch or clean requires a large repositioning of the feet, while the power snatch and power clean do not require such an adjustment.

In fixing the snatch overhead or the clean on the shoulders, the revolving Olympic-standard bar flips into its final receiving position. (See figure 4.7.) However, during this flip the bar normally again cuts back across the imaginary vertical line created when the bar was on the floor. Thus, you have performed a mild *S* pulling motion. This "hook" is more noticeable in the snatch than in the clean.

Recovery

Once the snatch or clean is securely in position, you stand up from the squat, split, or power position. (See figure 4.8.) When you and the barbell are motionless, the barbell is returned to the platform.

Basic Considerations

Nearly anyone can learn to efficiently execute a decent snatch or clean-and-jerk lift. These movements do not require unusual amounts of strength, power, flexibility, or coordination to perform. Without a doubt, proper practice will make these lifts easier, and thus more rewarding, to perform. Not only will you experience the pure satisfaction of performing a complex, ballistic, and total-body exercise, but you will also be able to apply these movements to those in your chosen sport.

However, not everyone comes to the platform with the same basic "equipment." Because the barbell remains pretty constant, other than how much it may weigh, what individual differences among athletes should be considered?

Grip

Let's start with the part of the body that will always be in contact with the barbell, the hands. Any athlete serious about achieving maximum performance will use what is called a "hook" grip. Although initially somewhat uncomfortable, this highly effective grasp on the bar should be used from day 1. The hook grip involves wrapping your index and middle fingers around the thumb, which is placed against the bar first. The ring and little fingers hold the bar rather loosely. (See figure 4.9.) This grip normally adds at least 10 percent to the amount lifted in any pulling motion. The hook grip is not used for pushing exercises.

FIGURE 4.9 Use of the hook grip is recommended for all pulling exercises.

Since the thumb takes a bit of a beating with the hook grip, most athletes wrap a short length of athletic trainer's tape around it. In official competition the tape may not cover the end of the thumb, but the actual length of tape is not measured.

When you first learn the movements with a dowel or empty bar, don't worry about taping your thumbs, but do use the hook grip. When you move up in weight beyond the empty bar, plan to wrap a piece of tape around that part of your thumb that comes in contact with the bar's knurling (the roughed-up part of the bar designed to facilitate a solid grip).

Your thumb's length is a factor in how effective the hook grip will be. Lifters with small hands or short thumbs often have trouble securing a solid hook grip, particularly for the snatch. Many lifters with short thumbs will release the hook grip once the bar is overhead in the snatch or on the chest in the clean.

Beginners often make the mistake of gripping the bar strongly with all fingers. In reality the grip, particularly in the snatch, consists mostly of the index and middle fingers, along with the thumb. The ring and little fingers remain in contact with the bar but do not have to be tightly gripped.

The cut of the knurling on some bars, or incorrect gripping, can lead to a common injury in weightlifters, a torn callus. It is important to keep calluses trimmed and neat, avoiding excessive torn skin in which chalk powder easily creeps. Sanding calluses is a regular ritual for most lifters. Don't lose training time because of a torn callus. Keep them sanded and ready for each workout.

Chalk

Magnesium carbonate or chalk, in block or powdered form, is a mainstay of a weightlifter's workout. As with gymnasts, chalk is applied liberally to the hands before nearly every pulling lift to provide a more secure grip. Chalk is available from a pharmacy or a sporting goods store.

It's a good idea to have something to keep the chalk in (a chalk box) to contain most of the chalk dust. Excess chalk on the floor does not endear weightlifters to most gym owners.

Straps

Straps are aids used to secure the grip for repetition snatches, cleans, or high pull exercises. (See figure 4.10.) Needless to say, straps greatly increase the amount of weight that can be lifted. Some athletes become dependent on such aids, which are not allowed in competition.

Straps can be made of several types of material, although cotton webbing seems the most comfortable, flexible, and forgiving on the wrists. Several construction designs are also available. An inexpensive means of creating a pair of straps is to purchase a cotton belt at a military surplus store. You don't need the buckle that is normally sold separately. Cut the brass tip off one end, fold the belt in half, and cut at the midpoint. Depending on your hand size, create two equal lengths about 14 to 18 inches long.

Be particularly careful using straps in the snatch. As we will soon discuss, having a barbell out of position, especially too far behind, requires you to safely drop the barbell to the platform. Dropping the bar from overhead (in

FIGURE 4.10   Pulling straps provide a more secure grip when performing many lifts.

front or behind) with straps tightly secured is not recommended. Most lifters learn through practice to open the hands, release the straps, and drop the bar safely. You should learn this action long before adding any significant weight to the bar.

Many athletes claim they cannot perform cleans with straps, but this seems related to poor flexibility of the wrists and shoulders.

Body Proportions

Just as hands and thumbs come in different sizes, so does the rest of the body. It is important to consider your individual build when deciding on a lifting style.

Arm Length

Elite weightlifters often have arms that are shorter than normal. This can be a real advantage in terms of how far the barbell must be lifted over the head. However, longer arms can be an advantage in lifting the bar from the floor because of a more favorable starting posture. The easiest way to determine your relative arm length is to take a "wing span test." Accurately measure your height against the wall, marking the top of your head. Place the middle finger of your left hand on this mark, turn your chest sideways to the wall, and reach to the floor with your right hand. Someone whose reach ("wing span") equals their height is considered to have normal-length arms; one whose arms are shorter than or longer than their height must learn to deal with that characteristic.

When you check photographs of lifters with the barbell overhead, most weightlifters (remember they tend to have short arms) have their elbows equal to or below the top of their head. Longer-armed individuals will often have their elbow joint located well above their head. Both Mitrou and Barnett excel in the jerk but due to the difference in arm length, note the difference in how far the bar is above their heads. (See figure 4.11.)

Leg Length

The overall length of the legs relative to the torso is important not only in terms of pulling positions, but also for receiving positions in the snatch or clean. Additionally, the ratio of the femur (thigh bone) to the tibia (shin bone) dictates much of the pulling or receiving positions a lifter will experience.

A lifter with a relatively short femur will not squat nearly as low to the floor compared to a lifter with a longer femur. Similarly, the starting position will vary greatly based on leg length. Although there is nothing you can do to change your body proportions, realize that champions come in all sizes and shapes. A knowledgeable coach can adjust your technique so that you can maximize your individual differences.

FIGURE 4.11 Victor Mitrou (GRE) and Wes Barnett (USA) both excel in the jerk despite differences in arm length.

Trunk Length

A lifter's trunk affects pulling and receiving postures. Kerri Hanebrink, with a long torso (see figure 4.12), shows a much different receiving position in the clean than Oscar Chaplin, with a short torso (figure 4.13). Torso length affects not only the receiving position, but also pulling positions. Lifters with a long femur (thigh bone) and short torso need to achieve excellent ankle flexibility to compensate, as shown by Szymon Kolecki (figure 4.14). In the initial stages of lifting a snatch or clean from the floor, a lifter with a long torso, or trunk, tends to position the shoulders farther in front of the bar than a lifter with a shorter torso. This affects how quickly the transition is made between the liftoff stage and the power position.

Also, assuming two lifters have similar upper-leg lengths, the lifter with the longer torso is more likely to keep his elbows clear of his knees in the squat clean position.

Equipment

You can benefit from performing explosive lifts with very basic barbell sets, but to maximize your efficiency and to make the activity safer and more comfortable,

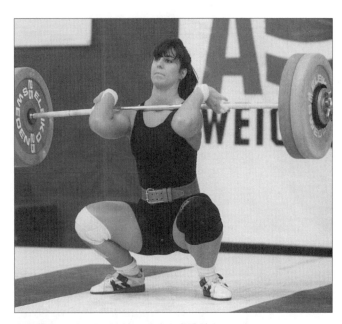

FIGURE 4.12 Kerri Hanebrink (USA) has a long torso, keeping her elbows clear of her knees.

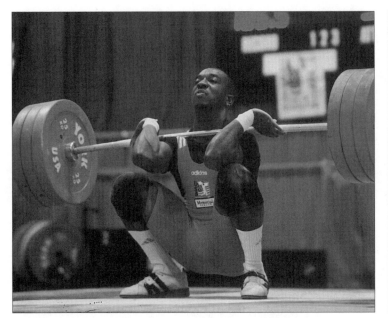

FIGURE 4.13 Oscar Chaplin's (USA) short torso brings his elbows in close proximity with his knees.

FIGURE 4.14 Szymon Kolecki (POL) keeps his elbows high despite having a short torso.

standard competitive weightlifting gear is the best choice. This includes not only what you lift but where you lift as well.

Don't get fooled into buying cheap, imitation equipment. Weightlifting training requires solid, well-constructed materials not found in the typical sporting goods store. Two barbells may appear at first glance to be identical, but the quality can vary greatly. Trying to save money by purchasing cheap materials will most likely lead to later problems and may seriously impact your safety.

Barbell

The most convenient barbell to use for weightlifting training is the so-called Olympic standard barbell. This name comes from the design approved by the International Weightlifting Federation, the governing body for international weightlifting.

The barbell unit consists of a bar, collars for securing weight plates or disks to the bar, and the actual weight plates. These consist of weights made up of 25, 20, 15, 10, 5, 2.5, and 1.25 kilograms. (The metric system is used extensively in weightlifting.) The size of the largest disk is 450 millimeters (18 inches) in diameter. As more and more athletes are drawn to weightlifting training, the full-size disks have become available in sizes down to 2.5 kilograms. This allows for a relatively light weight for learning technique while still allowing the barbell to have the same height from the floor that it would have with the heavier disks.

Another recent change in equipment has been the introduction of a bar designed for women competitors. The women's bar is 25 millimeters in diameter, compared to 28 millimeters for the men's bar. This allows for women's generally smaller hands to easily grasp the bar and perform lifts more comfortably.

Platform

In competition, the barbell and lifter are located on a platform that measures four meters square (about 13 feet on each side). Often, rubber inserts are placed in the wooden platform under the weights. This protects the platform and the weights from possible damage when the barbell is returned to the floor.

For training purposes, most lifters lift on a platform approximately eight feet square. Rubber inserts may be available as well.

In recent years special training platforms have become available that have incorporated the platform and rubber inserts, along with a "power rack," or multipurpose apparatus, from which to safely perform many assistance exercises.

Racks

The so-called power rack allows for safe execution of many exercises, even without a spotter. In addition, partial lifts or pulls can be performed from various heights. Other exercises to increase overhead stability may also be performed.

While it may be beyond the means of an individual training at home to have such an apparatus, these combination platforms and racks are available in high schools, colleges, and at fitness centers.

At the very least, someone training at home would require some form of squat rack, which could be simply two upright poles with a yoked top that holds the barbell. Alternatively, this may be a rack that allows for placement of the barbell at several different heights, thereby allowing different-size lifters to train together easily.

Clothing Requirements

The costume worn in weightlifting competition is referred to as a singlet. This is a highly specialized piece of wear not needed for the average athlete who simply uses weightlifting movements to improve sport performance. In most cases an athlete can easily get by with a simple shorts and T-shirt combination.

Since proper pulling technique calls for contact of the barbell on the thighs, it is a good idea to consider wearing sweatpants during most workouts. Maintain proper personal hygiene by carefully scrubbing with soap and water any abrasions that might occur from thigh contact with the bar.

Shoes are another highly specialized piece of equipment. These are specially designed to provide stability to the foot and to promote a solid footing on the platform while executing the lifts. For athletes using approximations of the snatch and clean-and-jerk movements (such as the power snatch and power clean), such specialized shoes are not necessary.

A weightlifting belt may be used, although its role is often overrated. The belt does not guarantee an injury-free experience, and in fact, its use most likely will keep the core musculature from becoming stronger. More on this later.

Supportive wraps worn around the knees and wrists, often seen in weightlifting competitions, do not need to be a concern for a beginner learning weightlifting movements. The wrist wraps, normally of elastic bandage quality, do help keep sweat from your hands while working out in a hot or humid environment. You are better off developing wrist flexibility than depending on wrist wraps to provide support. Knee wraps help keep the knee area warm and provide some support, but excessive dependence on this item may actually lead to knee injuries.

Safety

The actual performance of weightlifting exercises presents minimal risk, provided you learn proper technique and have professional supervision. However, you should take some steps to decrease the likelihood of being injured while weightlifting.

Spotting

Spotters are not used in weightlifting competition or training. It is the lifter's responsibility to safely drop a barbell that is out of position or results from a failed attempt. A spotter is much more likely to be injured than the lifter when lowering a barbell, so I absolutely discourage spotters for snatch and clean-and-jerk training.

As noted in chapter 9, spotters are required for certain assistance exercises such as the bench press and squat. For explosive weightlifting exercises, use the right equipment and learn to safely drop the barbell.

Collars

It is recommended that you always secure the plates to the bar with the use of appropriate collars. The collars will assure weights don't shift while you are lifting or fall off should you end up with the bar uneven overhead or on your chest. They only take a few seconds to use, so plan on including collars on each lift.

Dropping the Bar

Since the introduction of rubber "bumper" plates in the mid-1970s, the standard way to replace the barbell on the platform is to simply drop it (under control) from overhead. It seems the more experienced the athlete, the less likely they are to lower the barbell to its starting position. Dropping the bar, besides leading to possible damage to the weights and platform, is not without its own risks.

Depending on the total barbell weight and the dynamic of a particular brand of bumper plates, the bounce resulting from dropping the barbell to the platform can vary from a few inches to a couple of feet. This can be dangerous, particularly if the barbell bounces back toward your shins or knees.

For others in the immediate vicinity of the platform, a bouncing barbell can lead to injury. With some bumper plates, holding onto the bar and trying to absorb the bounce of the bumper plates can lead to wrist and hand injuries.

Early in the learning process you will be using very light weights to practice proper technique. In these workouts, practice lowering the barbell under complete control back to the platform. In a snatch-type movement this means performing an eccentric (negative) wide grip press until the bar is at about collarbone level. A quick flip of the elbows from under the bar to over the bar will then place the barbell below your waist. From here lower the bar either to the floor, the pulling blocks, or the hang position.

Lowering from the shoulders in the clean involves a quick flip of the bar and a reversal of elbow position from under the bar to over the bar. You then return the barbell to its starting position with the neutral spine position you used to lift initially.

The jerk is lowered slowly to the starting position on your shoulders. Your ankles, knees, and hips all flex slightly to absorb the weight as it is placed on your shoulders. Then, return the barbell to the rack or to the floor, depending on the starting position.

With additional weight on the bar, the process of lowering the barbell can become dangerous; in such situations the safest method is to simply drop the weights. The platform area must be kept free of objects, such as loose plates, collars, and so on. It is equally important that other lifters not be on the platform at the time.

In competition, lifters will most often keep their hands on the barbell until it is below the level of their waist. If the bar is dropped from that height, the best thing to do is step back slightly with both feet to avoid the bouncing barbell. In some instances experienced lifters appear to keep their arms straight as they let the bar fall to the platform. Since this is not a straight motion, but more of an arc, the resultant bounce of the bar can be unpredictable.

Losing the Bar Overhead

Despite the effort at perfecting technique, at times the bar will not be securely overhead (in the snatch or jerk) or on the chest (in the clean). In such instances it is important to know how to drop the bar safely.

Forward. When you fail to fix the bar overhead in the snatch and the bar is forward, you may have a tendency to try to step forward to "save" the lift. Within reason, this can work successfully, especially in a power snatch. If it happens in the bottom position of a squat snatch, a resulting "duckwalk" forward is *not* recommended. If by chance the bar is forward in a split snatch, again, you may be tempted to try to walk forward. In almost all instances, and particularly in a noncompetitive setting, this is *not* worth the effort. In these cases, simply hold onto the barbell and let it drop well in front of you (figure 4.15). Do not let go with the bar overhead, as the barbell will most likely bounce and roll forward off the platform, endangering others or equipment.

Backward. When the barbell drifts backward while overhead, it is almost always best to keep your elbows locked and allow the barbell to drop to the platform while you jump or step quickly forward (figure 4.16). Trying to hold onto a barbell drifting backward is almost always futile and may result in injury to your shoulders, elbows, or upper arms.

In a low split position, the loss of the barbell backward can be dangerous to your trailing leg. When this happens, quickly draw your rear leg forward, allowing the barbell to drop without contact.

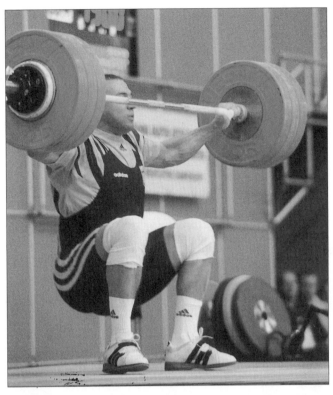

FIGURE 4.15 Denys Gotfrid (UKR) keeps his hands on the bar while safely dropping an out-of-position snatch.

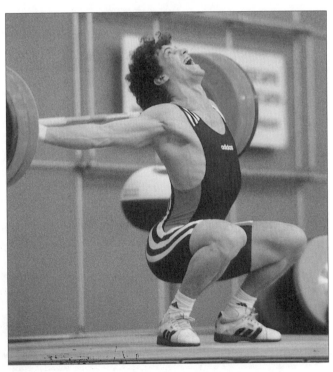

FIGURE 4.16 With good flexibility and straight arms, a failed snatch dropped behind presents no problem for Nikolai Peshalov (CRO).

In a power snatch, a simple step back may be sufficient to reposition your body under the bar, thus saving the lift, but this should not be exaggerated to involve more than a step.

In a power clean, a simple step backward may be sufficient to save the lift. Always be sure the area behind you is free of equipment or others so that you have adequate room to move if needed.

A squat clean with the bar moving backward cannot be saved through any means. It is possible to ascend from the bottom position and, once above parallel, step back; this is a very risky and difficult movement, however, and is not recommended. In the bottom position it is best to drop your hips backward while pushing the bar forward, resulting in your sitting down with the barbell on the platform in front of you.

On occasion, a rearward-moving barbell will take you back over onto your back with the bar still on your shoulders. With the use of full-size plates, the motion is not nearly as dramatic as weightlifting audiences often think. You are always safe, as the plates are high enough to pass over your face, after which you stand up.

In a lost jerk behind, your elbows cannot be kept straight because of your hand spacing on the bar. In this case it is important to drop the barbell quickly from the highest possible position, draw your rear leg forward, and step forward (figure 4.17).

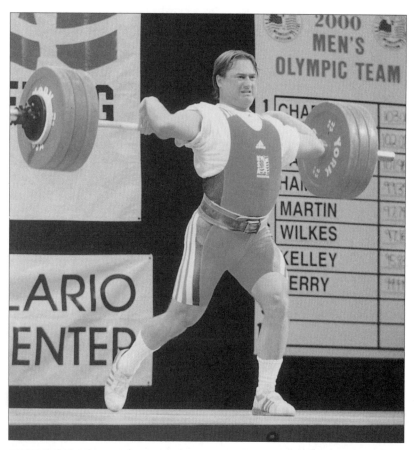

FIGURE 4.17 Pete Kelley (USA) steps forward from a jerk lost behind.

Practicing Losing the Barbell From Overhead

Although the previous strategies tend to all be safe, you cannot be expected to know how to drop the barbell safely without practice. You should practice safely dropping the barbell in different directions in the very early stages of learning to lift. These practice sessions *must* be performed with light weights. Such practice can come in extremely handy once heavier weights are loaded on the bar.

Remember that losing a lift is not a big deal. As in events like the high jump or pole vault, not every attempt will be successful, especially if appropriate loads are used. Missing a lift normally means that some technical error has occurred, and this can often be corrected on a subsequent lift.

Only competitive weight-lifters should truly experience missing a weight because the barbell is too heavy. Other athletes training with these movements normally do not need to handle loads that will lead to failure.

Everything I've talked about so far should give you a broad introduction to the various elements of explosive lifting. Now let's take a look at the specifics by beginning with the snatch.

Snatch

The snatch consists of rapidly lifting a barbell from its starting position on the floor to an overhead position in one continuous motion. An elite weightlifter can snatch a barbell weighing as much as double his body weight to arms' length in less than one second. This powerful movement is accomplished mostly through the use of the large muscles of the legs and hips, with the arms used only to quickly pull the body under the barbell and support the weight overhead. Of critical importance are the amount of power the lifter produces and how rapidly the lifter moves into receiving position.

Basic Snatch Styles

There are several different methods of snatch technique. Because of its popularity and relative ease of learning, I will reference the *squat* style for both the snatch and the clean throughout this book. The *split* style, while not seen to any great extent in competitive weightlifting arenas today, is a viable method of lifting greater weights than by simply using the power style. The *power* style of snatch and clean implies that the athlete has little interest in achieving maximum lift performance but still wants to gain the benefits of training in an explosive manner.

FIGURE 5.1   Squat Snatch

Squat Snatch

The squat snatch is the preferred manner for lifting the most weight in the snatch. After your legs and hips lift the weight from the floor, you execute a powerful jump, immediately followed by a pulling motion with your upper body and arms. With a sufficiently heavy weight, the barbell cannot be pulled completely overhead, so you actually pull yourself under the bar while the weight continues upward. The barbell arrives at arms' length about the time you arrive in a squat position under the bar. Stand up from the squat position to complete the lift. Ukraine's Timur Taimazov illustrates the squat snatch in figure 5.1.

a   Assuming a strong position.

b   Lifting off.

c   Bar at the knees.

d   Maintaining straight lift.

e   Scooping the knees and hips under the bar.

f   Explosive upward jump.

FIGURE 5.1 Squat Snatch

g   Maintaining upward momentum of bar.

h   Pulling body down.

i   Rotating the elbows forward.

j   Catching barbell at arm's length.

k   Initiating recovery.

l   Standing erect with the bar overhead.

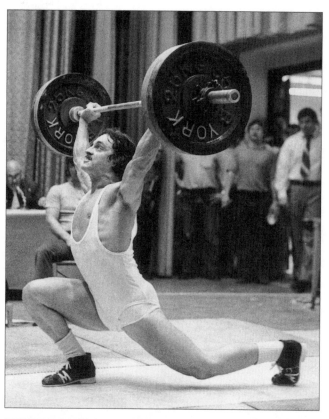

FIGURE 5.2   Al Stark (USA) performs a deep split snatch.

Split Snatch

Before the more efficient squat snatch technique was perfected, lifters used the split style. This requires a similar pulling motion, but at the height of the pull one foot is moved forward and the other rearward while still pulling the body underneath the barbell (figure 5.2). As we discussed earlier, you can't actually pull yourself against the barbell with your feet off the platform, and generally the split style requires your feet to remain in the air longer than in the squat style.

This style requires you to pull the bar a bit higher but results in a "catch" at arms' length similar to the squat style. Recovery to a standing position is accomplished by bringing your feet back in line. Although the split style has nearly disappeared from the competitive platform, it is quite easy to learn and has many applications for athletes of all sports, particularly those who use "lunge" positions similar to the split, such as ice hockey or tennis players.

Power Snatch

The power snatch is similar to the squat snatch, except you don't lower into a full squat position. Athletes with flexibility restrictions, particularly in the wrists, shoulders, lower back, hips, and ankles, may choose this style of snatching. Very tall athletes often have trouble performing the squat snatch either due to limitations on their grip width (even when collar-to-collar on the bar) or combined flexibility concerns. The power snatch is a suitable alternative.

The final receiving position for the power snatch is a half-squat with the barbell fixed overhead. Since the body is not lowered as far as in the squat snatch, the barbell must be lifted higher, so lighter weights are used. The power snatch is easy to learn and is a common part of the training program for weightlifters and athletes from other sports. Any strength or power athlete should benefit from the use of the power snatch.

Phases of the Snatch

The snatch, one of the most powerful athletic movements in sport, happens almost more quickly than the eye can follow. As a beginner, you may not be exactly sure how the bar gets overhead so quickly. Let's look at the essential stages any snatch lift passes through so that you'll understand what happens so quickly.

Starting Position

As we mentioned in chapter 4, a wide variety exists in the initial lifting posture. Using the squat style as a model, look at figure 5.1a for a solid starting position for the snatch. The feet are about hip-width apart, with the soles of the feet flat on the platform. The bar begins over the first metatarsal-phalangeal (MTP) joint of your feet. Bend your ankles, knees, and hips to lower your body to the bar, feeling your balance toward the front part of your foot. Use a wide, pronated (overhand) grip to grasp the bar. Remember, use the hook grip described in chapter 4.

Depending on your individual leverages, your hips should be approximately even with or just slightly higher than your knees, which should cause your shoulders to be over, or slightly in front of, the barbell. Rotate your elbows outward so that they are over the bar. Tuck your wrists slightly, retract your shoulder blades, and raise your chest. Keep your head in a neutral position, with your eyes focused directly ahead.

Liftoff

The initial movement is an extension of the hips and knees (figures 5.1b and c), which causes the bar to separate from the floor. Maintain the same torso angle throughout this part of the lift so that when the bar arrives at knee height, you have nearly the same angle between your hips and shoulders. Since the bar was directly over your toes before liftoff, the bar sweeps inward toward your shins a small distance. During this portion of the lift, your balance moves slightly from the front part of your foot to your midfoot.

Scoop

Your knees almost straighten completely but remain slightly bent. Further elevation of the bar now occurs by extending your hips. This means simply raising your shoulders vertically. The bar passes in front of your thighs until it reaches about midthigh, at which point you bring your hips to the bar. This movement results in a flexion of your ankles, knees, and hips, returning your balance to the front part of your foot (figures 5.1d and e). You have "scooped" your hips under the barbell, causing contact of the bar with the top of your thighs or your lower abdomen.

Jump

This is your "power position" (figure 5.1f), from which you now execute a powerful vertical jump that rapidly accelerates the bar upward (figure 5.1g). At the top of this movement, strongly contract the trapezius muscles of your upper back and begin to quickly bend your elbows, which remain over the barbell.

Pull-Under

The pull-under begins before the barbell loses its upward momentum (figure 5.1h). Understand that you can only accelerate your descent by pulling against the bar *with your feet on the floor*. Your wrists remain flexed, and the pulling effort is directed at rapidly lowering your own body weight under the bar. This is *not* a simple free fall maneuver.

Catch

Quickly rotate your elbows forward and push up against the bar, which is about to lose its upward motion and head downward (figures 5.1i and j). The actual catch, according to many-times World and Olympic champion Tommy Kono (USA), is felt in the wrists, which extend backward. The wrist, arm, and shoulder structure forms a solid line actively pushing up against the bar.

Recovery

Most lifters initiate their recovery from the squat position by extending their knees, pushing down against the floor, and allowing their hips to drift back slightly (figure 5.1k). This move requires excellent flexibility in the shoulders. After you get past the "sticking point" (about halfway up), bring your hips back under the barbell and stand up (figure 5.1l). If necessary, you can walk in any direction to gain full control of the barbell.

Learning the Snatch

The concept behind the snatch lift is relatively simple: stand up and squat down. Before trying the lift, however, let's determine the most effective grip placement and practice the receiving and recovery position. Once these preliminary steps feel comfortable, you'll be ready to start performing the snatch.

Grip Placement

Regardless of the style of snatch used, the initial steps are similar. The first step to learning the snatch is to determine the proper grip width. This is different for each lifter and is based on many variables, including thumb length and hand size, arm length, and shoulder flexibility.

In a classic squat snatch the bar is held at arms' length about four to eight inches above the head. This wide grip makes it easier to fix the bar overhead; plus, the bar does not have to be pulled very high before you descend under it. With a narrower grip, which requires more shoulder flexibility to place the bar overhead, you must pull higher. But this may be a more comfortable position, especially in the earlier stages. Much depends on the style of snatch used.

To determine your optimal snatch grip width, measure from the lateral (outside) head of the shoulder to the first knuckles of the closed fist of the opposite arm, which is abducted 90 degrees from the body (figure 5.3). The resulting distance is the correct measurement between the index fingers when you grip the bar to snatch (figure 5.4).

A grip this wide may take some getting used to. Beginners may wish to start with a slightly narrower grip, moving to the measured distance within a few weeks. Good flexibility of the wrist and shoulder joints is a must.

Press Behind the Neck

With the assigned grip in place, the first step is to practice a press behind your neck. You can choose to lift a dowel or an empty bar from the floor or

FIGURE 5.3 Grip measurement.

FIGURE 5.4 Grip placement.

take it from a squat or power rack. Rest the bar on your upper back (trapezius muscles), stand erect, and step back two to three steps from the rack. Keep your elbows directly under the bar while you press it overhead, then hold there for two seconds. (See figure 5.5 and 5.6.) This is the final receiving position for the snatch. It is important to keep your elbows under the bar and to extend your wrists fully so that your palms face toward the ceiling, not straight ahead.

Overhead Squat

Once you are comfortable holding the empty bar overhead with the proper grip, you're ready to move to the overhead squat. Should you decide to use the split-style snatch, this exercise is unnecessary, but you'll need to practice a lunge with the bar overhead to become accustomed to the split snatch receiving position.

FIGURE 5.5   Press behind neck start.

FIGURE 5.6   Press behind neck midpoint.

The overhead squat begins with the same first step as the press behind the neck. With the bar overhead, spread your feet to about shoulder-width, point your toes out slightly, and keep your feet flat on the floor (figure 5.7). Bend (flex) your ankles, knees, and hips to lower your body until the tops of your thighs are at least parallel to the floor. Keep your eyes focused straight ahead and maintain a rigid, but neutral, spine position (figure 5.8). This requires good flexibility in the lower back, hips, and ankles, in addition to the shoulders and wrists.

Pause for a moment in the bottom position, then recover to a standing position. If this feels comfortable, practice the overhead squat a few times, then rest. If you cannot attain this position easily, practice the squat without the bar, gradually getting into a comfortable squat position with your feet flat, your hips over your heels, and your spine flat and straight. Your torso should be nearly perpendicular to the floor. This could take several weeks of practice before you feel comfortable in a solid squat position.

Top-Down Learning Progression

While you could learn to snatch from the floor, this has its drawbacks. The most complicated part of the lift occurs toward the end of the pull, when the bar is moving fast. Since the simplest part of the pull is the initial pull from the floor, many coaches find it easier to teach the snatch from the top down, progressing from the most difficult stage to the easiest.

FIGURE 5.7   Overhead squat start.

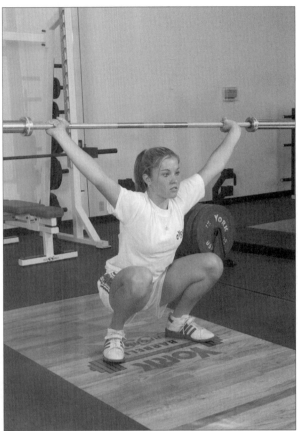

FIGURE 5.8   Overhead squat midpoint.

Regardless of the style of snatch you use, the actual process of pulling the bar overhead is nearly identical, so the top-down learning progression is suitable for all styles. Rather than squat or split during this learning process, feel free to keep your feet in place and execute a power snatch. I strongly suggest that you make your initial snatch efforts with no attempt to either jump off the floor or move your feet sideways. Remember, you want to learn what it feels like to pull yourself under the bar, and this can only be accomplished with your feet on the floor.

High Hang Snatch Pull

Whenever a snatch or clean is started from a position with the bar above the floor, we refer to this as "the hang." The top-down learning progression starts the lifting from the high hang position, just before the jump stage of the snatch pull. This is the so-called power position from which the most powerful vertical jump can be executed.

Many coaches encourage lifting from the hang position with little thought as to what this really means. It is not simply a matter of bending the ankles, knees, and hips a little bit, then exploding upward. To maximize your results, any hang must include the exact positions you pass through when lifting from the floor. Without careful attention to the subtle details of these positions, you may perform a snatch or clean in either power or full squat style but still miss the opportunity to develop maximum power.

FIGURE 5.9 **High Hang Snatch Pull**

Whether you take a dowel or empty bar from the floor or start with either object located on a stable set of blocks (figure 5.9a), get into position by dorsiflexing the ankles while flexing the hip and knee joints. Your arms are straight with the bar approximately at your hip joint. Your torso is flexed forward about 10 degrees. In this position your shoulders should be over or slightly in front of the bar. Your arms remain straight, the trapezius muscles

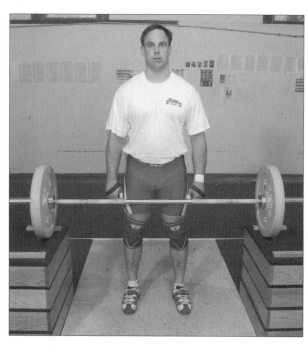

a   Position the barbell on blocks.

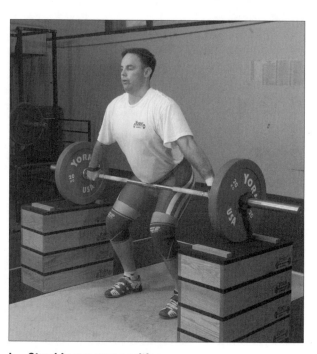

b   Stand in a power position.

c   Jump explosively upward.

d   Shrug and pull the barbell to sternum level.

of your upper back are stretched, your elbows are over the barbell, and your head is in a neutral position with your eyes focused straight ahead (figure 5.9b).

Initiate the pulling motion by rapidly extending your ankles, hips, and knees first, as in a vertical jump (figure 5.9c). Carry the barbell a short distance while it is in contact with your thighs or lower abdomen. Near the top of the jump quickly contract the trapezius muscles of your upper back. At this point pull your elbows up quickly but keep them over the bar. Your head stays in a neutral position with the line of sight straight ahead. Your entire body is stretched vertically, balanced on your toes (figure 5.9d). You should be able to hold this balanced position momentarily without losing balance forward or backward. When practicing this portion of the learning sequence, aim to pull the bar straight up your torso to a position equal to, or slightly higher than, your sternum. This requires good flexibility in your shoulder girdle.

You should make no deliberate attempt to hold this extended position. Lower the weight by straightening your elbows until the bar is back at the top of your thighs; then return your ankles, knees, and hips to the starting posture.

High Hang Power Snatch

You are now ready to enter the final stages of the lift. After successfully learning the high hang snatch pull, let's practice the full power snatch from the high hang. Once again, jump explosively upward (jump stage, figures 5.10a and b), pull the bar to about sternum height (figure 5.10c) *while at the same time* pulling yourself downward against the still-rising bar (pull-under stage). Your wrists remain flexed until the bar reaches the top of your head. With your feet firmly planted on the platform and your hips, knees, and ankles flexed, drive your elbows forward and under the bar (catch stage, figure 5.10d). At this stage you push yourself against the bar until your elbows lock out the bar overhead (figures 5.10e and f).

You've lowered your body about 6 to 10 inches into a partial squat and now have the bar at its final position overhead. Hold this position for one to three seconds; then straighten your ankles, knees, and hips to recover to a standing position (recovery stage).

Timing the end of the pull is an important skill that requires coordination and experience. Since the snatch cannot end with a "press out," this catch phase must occur quickly and without hesitation. A press out is a technical rules violation that indicates the barbell did not go immediately to arms' length. If you catch the barbell overhead with flexed (bent) elbows and press the bar to arms' length, you've performed a press out. This problem is normally avoided by pulling adequately high and lowering rapidly to a locked out (elbows straight) position.

At this stage of learning, your feet should remain in the same position throughout. Don't jump off the floor or move your feet to the sides.

To lower the bar from overhead, slowly bend your elbows and "reverse press" the weight toward your shoulders. When the bar reaches about the level of your face, flip your elbows over quickly and lower the bar to the original starting position. This final stage is accomplished by once again flexing your ankles, knees, and hips to absorb the descending bar.

FIGURE 5.10 High Hang Power Snatch

a   Assume the power position.

b   Jump explosively upward.

c   Shrug and pull the bar upward.

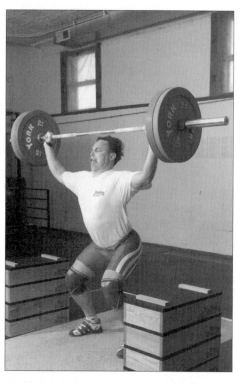

d   Maintain bar momentum and pull your body under the bar.

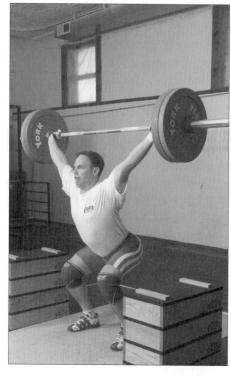

e   Lock out bar overhead with straight arms.

f   Recover to a standing position.

This is the power position that will create explosive strength in the Olympic-style lifts. This violent vertical jump action imparts the impetus to the bar that makes these lifts so challenging and rewarding. Some athletes may never have a need to snatch from any position other than this one to benefit from this type of training.

FIGURE 5.11   Low Hang Snatch Pull

Low Hang Snatch Pull

After several workouts of snatching successfully from the high hang position, the next phase calls for the bar to be lowered to a position just below your knees. We'll start by performing only the pulling stage of the lift from this position.

Place the bar just below your kneecaps, with your knees slightly flexed, your torso rigid and spine neutral, and your shoulders over the bar (figure 5.11a). Your ankle joints are nearly open, with only about 5 degrees of flexion. You should feel a considerable stretch in your hamstrings while in this

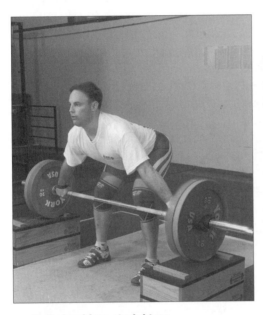

a   Pull shoulders straight up.

b   Scoop into power position.

c   Jump explosively upward.

d   Shrug and pull bar to sternum level.

73

position; successful execution of this lift requires excellent flexibility. Your balance is located around the middle of your foot. Your arms remain straight, and your elbows are locked and over the bar. Your neck is in a slightly extended position with your eyes focused straight ahead or at the end of the platform. Do not look toward the ceiling.

Through hip extension, your shoulders rise straight up until the bar is at about midthigh level. As the bar passes your midthigh, your ankles quickly dorsiflex, resulting in a flexion of your knees and hips. The lowering of your hips results in the bar contacting your upper thighs or lower abdomen as in the high hang posture (figure 5.11b).

From here you execute the pull as previously learned (figure 5.11c), finishing with the bar under your chin and your elbows pointed straight up (figure 5.11d). Although this complicated maneuver requires a relatively slow learning speed, it is imperative that the motion is continuous and that maximum speed is used as soon as possible. This scooping action allows your lower body to get into position to actually *push* the bar overhead, while your upper body *pulls* the bar to its final position. Finally, lower the bar as before to the starting position and repeat the lift.

It is much easier and more consistent to use special pulling blocks to achieve the same bar position for each repetition. Most beginners find this portion of the snatch difficult to learn, as they tend to depend on the strong hip extension alone to raise the weight, avoiding bar contact with the thighs. You can get away with this if you're lifting only an empty bar or a light weight, but if you want to ultimately lift heavier weights, this scooping action must be learned as one continuous motion.

It is crucial to quickly and successfully flex your ankles, knees, and hips to get into the power position. As discussed in chapter 3, this amortization phase of the stretch-sequence cycle must reverse direction quickly to maximize the plyometric effect. It will take many workouts before you successfully and consistently execute this motion. However, it is essential that you learn this phase properly, slowly at first, but then with maximum speed.

Low Hang Power Snatch

From the same starting position (figure 5.12a), you pull the bar to the power position (figure 5.12b), explode vertically (figure 5.12c), and pull yourself under the rising bar (figure 5.12d) as you did from the high hang position. Focus on lifting your shoulders straight up and scooping your hips under the bar; then execute a big vertical jump, followed by aggressively pulling yourself under the bar (figure 5.12e). Stand up (figure 5.12f), lower the weight from overhead, and set up for the next repetition.

From the Floor

Now that the fastest and most difficult stages have been learned, place the barbell on the platform. Since you have learned the more complicated later stages of the lift, this first part (lifting the bar from the floor to about your knees) will be relatively simple to learn.

The liftoff begins with your feet flat; your ankles, knees, and hips flexed; your torso flexed; and your shoulders over the bar. Your elbows are fully extended and over the bar, with your center of balance toward the front part of your foot (figure 5.13a on page 76).

FIGURE 5.12   Low Hang Power Snatch

a   Pull shoulders straight up.

b   Scoop into power position.

c   Jump explosively upward.

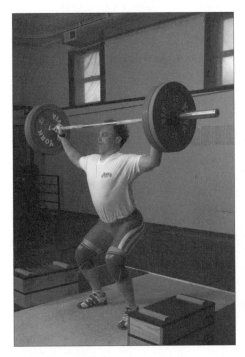

d   Shrug and pull under rising bar.

e   Catch at arms' length.

f   Recover to standing position.

FIGURE 5.13   Power Snatch From the Floor

a   **Starting position.**

b   **Lift bar to below the knees.**

c   **Scoop into power position.**

d   **Jump explosively upward.**

e   **Maintain upward momentum of the bar.**

f   **Pull under bar and catch at arms length.**

Through a combined extension of your knees and hips ("pushing the floor away"), raise the bar to a position just below your knees (figure 5.13b). Remember from chapter 4 that the initial liftoff is not performed in a perfectly straight line, but the bar moves slightly toward your shins while simultaneously moving upward. At the same time your center of balance shifts slightly rearward to the center of your foot (see figures 5.13c-f).

The remainder of the lift is executed as previously rehearsed from the low hang and high hang positions.

Now that you've become familiar with executing the power snatch, it's time to start the process over, using the squat or split receiving position, depending on your preference.

Mastering the power snatch first keeps you focused on getting the bar quickly overhead. With the introduction of the squat or split, you may find that your balance is a factor. Patiently practice the same system of progression and drill many, many repetitions with the empty bar or dowel. You want to establish a motor pathway that allows for consistent execution during every repetition. As soon as your technique becomes established, focus on gaining greater speed.

Only after you can consistently and quickly perform the full snatch with a dowel, empty bar, or light barbell, should you consider moving up in resistance. Maintain the quality of each repetition and don't concern yourself with the amount of weight used. That comes later.

Pulling Blocks

The various stages of the snatch can be learned by simply holding the bar in the desired position (power position, at the knees, on the floor) or from special pulling boxes or blocks. The latter allow the bar to regain its exact starting position each repetition, in addition to allowing you to relax or regrip the bar each repetition. Blocks can be easily built or purchased.

Keep in mind, however, that performing any pulling motion from the blocks while in an incorrect position may interfere with the proper learning of the complete movement. It takes a great deal of insight to know how to duplicate exactly your personal best power position or pull from your knees. Seek the assistance of a highly qualified coach when performing lifts from the blocks.

The blocks introduce an additional obstacle to the combined lifter-barbell-platform environment. Beginners with several months' experience can safely use the blocks for light to moderate full snatches or cleans, or heavier high pull exercises. Only skilled and experienced lifters should consider using the blocks for heavy full attempts.

Take your time and learn each step of the snatch progression. Only after you consistently demonstrate correct positions, speed, and balance should you gradually and systematically introduce heavier weights. Learning the snatch will prepare you for the next lift, the clean.

Clean

The clean is the first stage of the two-part competitive lift, the clean-and-jerk. The clean requires lifting the barbell from the floor to a final resting position across the anterior deltoids (shoulders) and clavicles (collarbones). The pulling portion of the clean is a very rapid movement, with the bar normally placed on the shoulders in less than one second. In the lighter body weight categories, elite male weightlifters have lifted triple their body weight in the clean-and-jerk. Elite females have surpassed double their body weight.

Basic Clean Styles

Like the snatch, the clean has several varieties that may be performed. Since the *squat clean* is the most popular version of the lift, this will be our point of reference in this chapter. The *split clean*, although no longer used much on the competitive weightlifting platform, remains a viable method of lifting heavier weights than can be handled in the power clean. The *power clean* is a simple way to get the barbell to the shoulders and is the most common form of the clean in resistance training programs for strength and power athletes. Its application in competitive weightlifting is quite limited, although it remains a popular and effective training exercise.

FIGURE 6.1   Squat Clean

Squat Clean

The squat clean is the preferred manner for lifting the most weight to your shoulders. As in the snatch, the large muscles of your legs and hips are used to lift the barbell from the floor. The bar moves continually upward while you shift into position to perform a powerful jump combined with an explosive pulling motion with your upper body and arms. You aggressively pull yourself into a squat position to catch the bar. This catch, or rack, occurs by quickly rotating your elbows under the bar. A smoothly executed clean allows you to rapidly recover from the low squat position and stand to complete the lift. Pete Kelley (USA) performs the squat clean in figure 6.1.

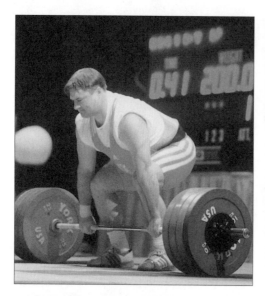

a   **Assuming a strong position.**

b   **Strong liftoff with knee and hip extension.**

c   **Lifting, maintaining torso angle.**

d   **Lifting straight up.**

FIGURE 6.1   Squat Clean

e   **Jumping explosively upward.**

f   **Shrugging and pulling down.**

g   **Solidly racking the bar.**

h   **Deep squat clean position.**

i   **Recovery by easing hips to the rear.**

j   **Standing to complete the clean.**

Split Clean

In the early days of competitive weightlifting most lifters used the split clean to get heavy weights onto their shoulders. This style is seldom seen in present-day competitions, but the split clean does provide a reasonable way for many athletes to lift greater weights to their shoulders. As in the snatch, this style has direct application for athletes who participate in sports that require a lunge position.

The pull in the split clean is nearly identical to the pull in the squat style, but near the maximum height of the pull, you step one foot forward and the other one rearward. Pull yourself underneath the barbell as the weight is racked, as in the squat clean. As previously discussed, you cannot actually pull against the bar if your feet are off the floor. Since the split clean requires your feet to be airborne, the pull must be higher than the pull for the squat clean. The split itself should be wide and deep, with your front thigh parallel to the floor and your front knee over your front foot. (See figure 6.2.) Your rear leg is nearly straight, with your balance maintained by your toes, which are dorsiflexed. You then recover to a standing position to complete the clean.

Untrained novices in the weight room sometimes perform a shallow split clean accomplished by shuffling their feet a short distance or only moving one foot rearward. This action really does not allow you to lower your body under the bar sufficiently to warrant the use of a split. Instead of a partial split clean, you are much better off performing a power clean.

Power Clean

The pulling action for the power clean is similar to that for the squat clean. The final position to catch or "rack" the bar is much different, however. You again bend your hips, knees, and ankles and lower your body but only to a partial squat position. Since your body is not lowered as far as in the squat clean, the bar must be raised higher; this limits the amount of weight you can lift. As with the power snatch, a longer, higher pull for the power clean may compromise the explosive benefit of this exercise. If you decide to train with the power clean instead of the squat clean, focus on quick execution, and don't concentrate on pulling excessively high.

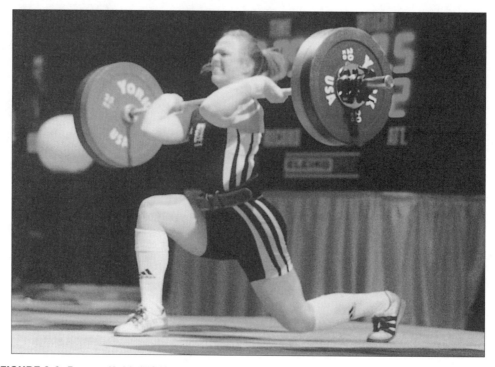

FIGURE 6.2 Doreen Heldt (USA) cleans with a strong, deep split.

The power clean is simple to learn and generates a lot of power. This combination makes the power clean very popular with athletes and coaches of many sports. It can be especially helpful for athletes whose flexibility or limb lengths do not allow them to get into a comfortable front squat position, a requirement for a successful squat clean.

As popular as the power clean is in most programs, far too many athletes don't perform the lift properly. Lack of solid support for the bar on the shoulders and collarbones can lead to hand or wrist injuries. Jumping the feet excessively to the sides rather than flexing the ankles, knees, and hips can lead to lower-extremity injury and instability. Racking the bar with a rounded upper back can easily injure the back.

Phases of the Clean

Most of the characteristics of the clean are similar to those of the snatch, except of course that the bar does not go overhead. Most athletes find the clean considerably easier to master than the snatch, since placing the bar on the shoulders rather than overhead encourages greater stability and balance.

Starting Position

As we will soon see, the suggested grip for the clean is considerably closer than that for the snatch. This narrower grip allows you to place your torso in a more upright starting position, which feels more efficient. Because your torso is more erect, your hips can also be placed somewhat higher than in the snatch. Your feet may be placed a bit closer to the bar than for the snatch. All of these details should allow for a more comfortable starting position and stronger liftoff.

Place your feet under the bar so that the bar appears directly over the first laces of your lifting shoes, or about the widest portion of your foot. Foot spacing is again about hip-width apart, with your toes pointed either straight ahead or slightly outward. Once your feet are set, flex your ankles, knees, and hips and squat down until your thighs are about parallel to the floor. Keep your shoulders slightly in front of the bar and feel your balance on the front part of your foot. Using the hook grip, grasp the bar, rotate your elbows outward, and lock them. Inflate your chest, lock your spine into a neutral position, and look straight ahead or slightly downward.

Liftoff

Once again, the initial muscular action that separates the barbell from the platform is an extension of your knees and hips (figure 6.1a and b). This allows the bar to rise with a slight sweep toward your shins, which also causes your balance to shift to the middle of your foot. Do not allow yourself to shift this balance farther back than midfoot.

As you "push the platform away," concentrate on lifting your shoulders straight up. You should perform this liftoff strongly, without hesitation. However, be very careful not to rush the knee extension, which will cause the common newcomer problem of the knees straightening before the hips, thus causing the torso angle to drop. This error results in other problems later in the lift.

Scoop

Because of more favorable leverage in the clean, you can keep the bar clear of your thighs as you continue to lift the bar by means of hip extension. This requires an extremely strong set of spinal erector muscles, along with excellent hamstring strength and flexibility. Continue lifting your shoulders straight up until the bar reaches about midthigh, when your hips are driven toward the bar (figure 6.1c and d). By keeping your feet flat on the platform, the forward hip drive results in a bending of your ankle, knee, and hip joints under the bar. Be sure to keep your arms perfectly straight. Depending on your grip width, individual leverages, and general technique, the bar should contact your thighs from midthigh up to your hip joint. At this point, keep your shoulders over the barbell as long as possible.

Jump

With feet flat and ankles, knees, and hips slightly flexed, you are coiled and ready to perform a powerful vertical jump. Jump explosively upward, but do not try to jump off the floor. In the clean, the bar is not pulled higher than your navel. But before the momentum of this powerful jump drops off, violently contract your trapezius (upper-back) muscles and bend your elbows as you begin to pull yourself under the bar (figure 6.1e).

Pull-Under

If you have kept your elbows over the bar as you should have, the bar will be very close to your torso. The shrugging motion of your upper back, coupled with a very aggressive arm flexion will accelerate your body downward against the barbell (figure 6.1f). Again, this cannot be accomplished properly if your feet are off the floor. If you have to reposition your feet for better receiving position, keep them close to the plateform. Don't relax or free fall during this part of the lift.

Rack

The bar still has some momentum carrying it upward, so it is important that you coordinate receiving the bar on your shoulders. The Olympic standard bar revolves easily as you rotate your elbows forward and under the bar. Your wrists extend as your shoulders are raised slightly to cushion the landing of the bar. Your elbows need to be high enough to avoid any contact with your thighs or knees (figure 6.1g). Not only is elbow contact with the thighs or knees a technical rules violation (not a "clean" lift), but this may also lead to a serious wrist injury.

Once the weight is racked, you ride the bar down into squat position (figure 6.1h). Be sure to grip the bar completely with your hands; don't let it roll onto just your fingertips. Maintain a flat and rigid torso, with your chest high. Plan to spend the least amount of time necessary in the bottom position of the squat.

Recovery

Standing up from the squat position will vary greatly in effort based on your leg strength, flexibility, timing, and the overall smoothness of the clean. Push your elbows up to keep the bar in its racked position and keep your chest inflated and in front of the bar. Many lifters allow their hips to drift back slightly as they work through the "sticking point," or the most difficult biomechanical position when the thighs are approximately parallel to the floor (figure 6.1i). If your hips drift back excessively, your torso angle will drop, making it impossible to hold the bar in position.

Rise from the bottom squat position with your hips over your heels and your torso inclined forward only a very small amount. After you get through the sticking point, be sure to keep your hips under the bar and your torso erect (figure 6.1j).

Learning the Clean

Learning how to perform a clean successfully is a fairly easy task. It is crucial that you focus on linking together the correct movements to learn the proper technique. Don't try to "muscle up" the weight by using your arms (easily accomplished with light instructional weights). Work on the development of a smooth technique, using your body effectively to ultimately lift much heavier weights.

Grip Placement

Determining where to grip the bar depends on the size and flexibility of the athlete. Like the snatch grip, the clean grip varies with the individual needs of the lifter. The technical rules allow for a modification of the grip between the clean and the jerk should you prefer to change grip width after cleaning the weight.

The clean-and-jerk calls for a grip a little wider than your shoulder-width. (See figure 6.3.) Start by placing your index fingers near the edge of the bar's knurling. Experiment with moving your grip out from this starting point. For most athletes, a comfortable grip about a thumb's length from the bar's smooth section will be optimal for both the clean and the jerk. Pulling with this width grip allows the bar to contact your legs at about midthigh level when in the power position.

During the initial stages of learning the clean you must become accustomed to holding the bar solidly on your shoulders. Since this is the final position for the clean and the beginning position for the jerk, a stable position is crucial. Due mostly to a lack of flexibility, many novices experience difficulty keeping their hands closed while resting the bar on their shoulders. Although some coaches allow or encourage an athlete to open his hand, thus resting the bar on his fingertips, this should be discouraged for most lifters.

It is better to take the extra time to develop the necessary flexibility required to secure the bar properly. This will require flexibility in your wrists, elbows, triceps, shoulders, and upper-back region. Continued holding of the

FIGURE 6.3   The clean grip is slightly wider than your shoulders.

bar in the proper position will aid flexibility. Once this position becomes comfortable (and this may take a few weeks), you are ready to progress to the front squat.

Front Squat

The front squat is introduced once you can easily hold the bar in the proper position with a completely closed hand and you have achieved the desired squatting position. If you have problems with a proper squat position, improve this first before using the bar. Proper squatting or front squatting requires a flat back and erect posture, with your feet flat on the platform. Your ankles, hips, and lower back all must be flexible to achieve this correct position.

Place a bar at about shoulder height in a squat or power rack. Grip the bar with an overhand (pronated), closed grip, and rotate your elbows under the bar as you step under the bar with both feet. Your elbows are placed about halfway between perpendicular to the floor and horizontal to the floor, pointed slightly outward.

Keep your torso nearly perpendicular to the floor (a very slight forward incline is permitted), and take and hold a deep breath as you lift the bar from the rack. After gaining balance and control, step backward out of the rack area two paces. Exhale, fix your line of sight on a position at approximately eye level, and again inhale, holding this breath (figure 6.4).

Flex (bend) your ankle, knee, and hip joints so that your body descends to a position where the tops of your thighs are at least parallel to the floor. (See figure 6.5.) Return to a standing position, exhaling as your body rises.

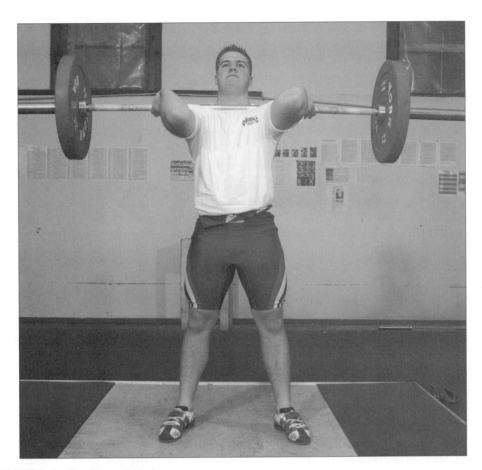

FIGURE 6.4   Front squat start.

FIGURE 6.5   Front squat midpoint.

Repeat for the desired number of repetitions, then return the bar to the squat rack by stepping forward two steps. Check the bar/rack alignment before lowering the bar to its final resting position.

Once you can perform the front squat correctly, you're ready to move on to learning how to clean. The following learning sequence is designed to use with the squat clean. If you cannot squat properly, don't automatically focus on the power clean. Novices often tend to use sloppy posture in catching the bar when doing a power clean. Rather than lowering the body to a half-squat position, beginners often resort to leaning back or jumping excessively sideways, both of which can lead to unnecessary injury.

You should work at hitting the correct front squat position before learning the clean. If it just isn't going to happen, plan to learn the split clean. The sequence for learning the split clean is identical to that for the squat clean.

Top-Down Learning Progression

As with the snatch, you can learn to perform the clean from the floor, but I think it's easier to employ the top-down learning progression, learning the later, more difficult maneuvers first. Again, regardless of whether you plan to use the squat, split, or power clean, the learning sequence is identical. Should you decide to use the split or power clean varieties, however, you should be aware that the recovery description offered here is appropriate only for the squat clean. If you split clean, recover using the sequence taught in the next chapter for the split jerk. The power clean requires only that you stand up from the semi-squat position where you racked the bar.

High Hang Clean Pull

To learn the clean, start in the "power position." This is the position from which the most powerful vertical jump can be executed (figure 6.6a). This means a dorsiflexion of your ankle joints, along with a slight flexion of your hip and knee joints. The balance is toward the front part of your foot.

The bar is at arms' length, resting approximately at midthigh (this will depend on the length of your arms, the width of your grip, and your arm-torso-leg proportions). Keep your torso flexed at the waist about 5 to 10 degrees. Position your shoulders over or slightly in front of the bar. Your arms are straight, the trapezius muscles of your upper back are stretched, your elbows are over the barbell, and your head is neutral with your eyes focused straight ahead.

It is important to initiate the pulling motion by explosively extending your ankles, knees, and hips, as in a vertical jump. Don't contract your trapezius muscles or your arms prior to jumping. Carry the barbell for a short period of time while it is in contact with your thighs (figure 6.6b). As you complete the jump (figure 6.6c), strongly contract your trapezius muscles and move your elbows upward sharply, keeping your elbows and shoulders over the bar (figure 6.6d).

Don't make a deliberate attempt to hold this extended position, but instead return your elbows to a straight position; lower the bar back to your midthighs; and flex your ankles, knees, and hips to return to the starting posture.

FIGURE 6.6 High Hang Clean Pull

a   The bar starts at midthigh.

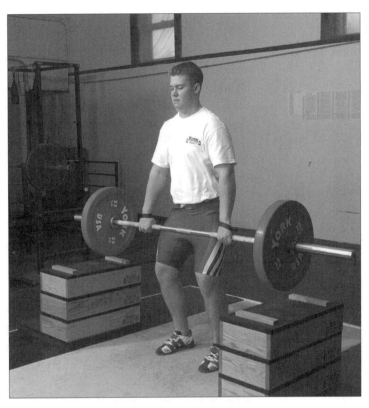

b   Carry the bar while jumping explosively upward.

c   Reach triple extension of ankles, knees, and hips.

d   Shrug and pull the bar to about navel height.

High Hang Squat Clean

Now you are ready to enter the final stage of the pull that results in your actually cleaning the bar (figure 6.7a). As before, your explosive upward jump causes the bar to travel several inches above your navel, while at the same time you initiate a strong downward pull against the still-rising bar (figure 6.7b and c). Keep your wrists flexed until the bar reaches breastbone height. Flex your knees and ankles as your body lowers under the bar.

Excellent timing is needed to successfully move your elbows rapidly in front of the bar while extending your wrists and having the revolving bar re-orient to its landing position on your shoulders and collarbones. This phase occurs quickly and without hesitation (figure 6.7d). You will need lots of practice to avoid the common fault of letting the bar "crash" into its final position. "Crashing" occurs when you either overpull (pull too high) the bar or drop too fast or too far under the bar before properly racking the bar on your shoulders and collarbones.

As the bar reaches its final position on your shoulders, your body is 6 to 8 inches into the squat position. Continue to descend to the bottom squat position with the bar in place on your shoulders, then start the recovery by lifting against the bar while straightening your ankles, knees, and hips until you are standing erect.

Lower the bar by flipping the bar off your shoulders and catching it at the top of your thighs with a slight bend of your knees and ankles.

What has just occurred is cleaning from the high hang position. This is the power position so crucial to success in the Olympic-style lifts and beneficial for athletes of many different sports.

Low Hang Clean Pull

After several workouts of successful cleans from the high hang position, the next phase calls for you to lower the bar to a position approximately at your knees.

It is usually best to position the bar just below your kneecaps, with your knees slightly flexed, your torso rigid, and your shoulders forward of the bar. Your ankle joints are nearly straight, with up to about 5 degrees of flexion. The balance is felt on the middle of your foot. Your arms remain straight, and your elbows are locked and directly over the bar. Your neck is in a slightly extended position with your eyes focused straight ahead (figure 6.8a on page 92).

As in the snatch from the low hang position, the pull from this position is initiated with a strong hip extension. The bar rises to about midthigh level as your shoulders lift straight upward (figure 6.8b). With the bar around midthigh level and still rising, you dorsiflex your ankles, resulting in a flexion of your knees and hips (figure 6.8c). The rapid scoop or lowering of your lower body results in the bar contacting your thighs as practiced in the high hang posture.

From here you execute the lift as previously learned. (See figure 6.8d and e.) Lower the bar as before, back to the starting position, and then repeat.

Starting with the bar around your knees is the most difficult phase to learn. As in the snatch, later progress is contingent on successfully mastering the manipulation of your body into the power position. This phase, with the lowering of your hips into the power position, may take many

FIGURE 6.7 **High Hang Squat Clean**

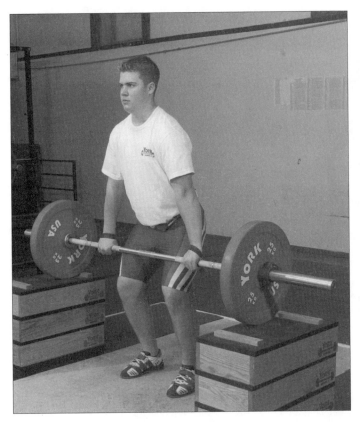

a   Bar is at midthigh.

b   Jump explosively upward.

c   Shrug and pull under the rising bar.

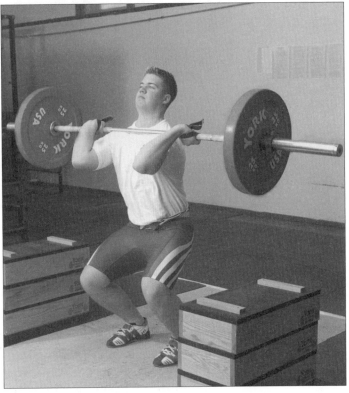

d   Rack solidly and descend to the squat position.

FIGURE 6.8 Low Hang Clean Pull

a Bar starts just below the knees.

b Raise your shoulders straight up.

c Scoop by bending ankles, knees, and hips.

d Jump explosively upward.

e Shrug and pull the bar to navel height.

workouts to execute successfully. However, it is essential to master this phase properly. Start performing this pull slowly at first, but as soon as you can consistently execute the movement, perform it with increased speed in order to maximize the plyometric effect.

Low Hang Squat Clean

After you have successfully mastered the pulling motion for below your knees (and this may take several workouts), you're ready to move to the clean from the low hang. This builds on movements already mastered.

From the low hang position (figure 6.9a) you initiate the pulling motion as previously learned, placing the bar at midthigh level (figure 6.9b) and jumping explosively upward. Before the upward momentum of the bar drops off, smoothly and aggressively pull your body downward against the bar

FIGURE 6.9 Low Hang Squat Clean

a Bar starts just below the knees.
b Raise shoulders straight up and scoop.
c Jump explosively upward.

d Shrug and pull down against rising bar.
e Rack solidly on shoulders.

f Descend to squat clean position.
g Recover to a standing position.

(figure 6.9c). Time the rack properly (figure 6.9d and e), absorbing the weight of the bar, descend to the squat position (figure 6.9f), then return to the standing position (figure 6.9g). Flip the bar off your shoulders, absorb the descending bar with bent knees and arms, and place the bar back in its starting position. Repeat for the desired number of repetitions.

Continue to practice this movement until all the segments fit together easily and you can perform a well-coordinated, explosive lift without hesitation.

From the Floor

With the most difficult phase now successfully mastered, let's move to the full lift with the barbell on the floor. Having learned the more complicated maneuvers already, the first part of the lift (the bar rising from the floor to a position around your knees) will be relatively simple to learn.

The liftoff begins with your feet flat; your ankles, knees, and hips flexed; your torso flexed; and your shoulders over the bar (figure 6.10a). Your elbows are fully extended and over the bar. Take in a full breath before lifting and force your chest up and forward. Your center of balance is toward the front part of your foot.

Through a combined extension of your knees and hips ("pushing the floor away"), raise the bar to a position just below your knees (figure 6.10b). Now perform the clean as previously rehearsed. (See figure 6.10c through f.)

As we discussed in chapter 5, these various pulling stages can be learned by simply holding the bar in the desired position (power, at the knees, on the floor) or from special pulling boxes or blocks. While I am a very strong proponent of learning the lifts from the blocks, I recognize that the exact positions may not be practiced. This mistake can lead to a lot of later frustration, so if you use blocks, carefully check your positions and enlist the best coaching help available.

Now let's move on to the jerk. It is a quick, compact movement while at the same time being complex and requiring attention to detail.

FIGURE 6.10 Squat Clean From the Floor

a Strong starting position.

b Liftoff with knee and hip extension.

c Maintain torso angle.

d Scoop and jump explosively upward.

e Shrug and pull down against the rising bar.

f Rack solidly on shoulders, descend, and recover.

7

Jerk

After you have successfully cleaned the barbell, all that remains is to quickly "jerk" the weight overhead. This relatively simple movement often determines the winner in a weightlifting contest, which is why the clean-and-jerk is known as the King of Lifts.

Like the snatch, the jerk is executed so quickly that many newcomers can't comprehend how the lift occurred. This multiple-joint lift gains most of its impetus from the strength and power of the lower body. The arms and shoulders only push the body under the rising bar and hold it in the final position. Weights two to three times body weight are regularly lifted in the jerk.

Basic Jerk Styles

Until fairly recently, there was really no variation in jerk styles. Nearly everyone performed the traditional split jerk. However, now we see several different forms of jerk technique successfully used at the international level of competition. Strength coaches find it helpful to introduce athletes to all varieties, which we will do in this chapter.

FIGURE 7.1   Split Jerk

Split Jerk

All forms of the jerk lift involve a short bend and powerful extension of the legs to push the bar off the shoulders, followed by lowering the body, securely fixing the weight overhead, and recovery to a standing position. Nearly all weightlifters employ the split jerk technique. Because of its safe, simple, and secure format, the split jerk is the only technique necessary for the beginner to learn. Olympic gold medalist Tara Nott (USA) jerks heavy weight over her head in figure 7.1.

After performing a successful clean, catch your breath and prepare mentally and physically for the jerk. A rapid, but controlled, flexion of your ankle, knee, and hip joints causes your body to descend about four to six inches into a quarter-squat position. You then quickly reverse direction, just as in jumping, and push upward. As the bar clears your shoulders, split your legs by placing one foot forward and one rearward. During this very fast action you lower your body to receive the bar overhead. Once the bar is secure, recover to a standing position and return the bar to the platform.

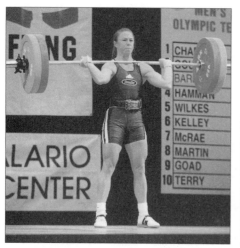

a   Tara Nott (USA) prepares to jerk.

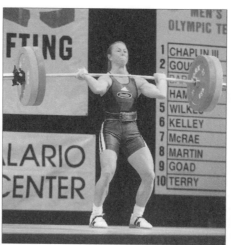

b   Bending knees, ankles, and hips to descend.

c   Jumping explosively upward.

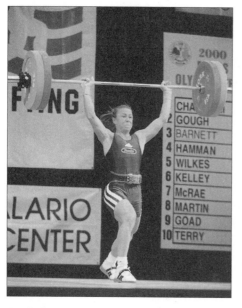

d   Split feet while pushing against bar.

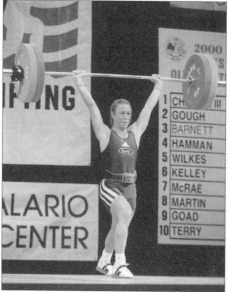

e   Catching the bar at arms' length.

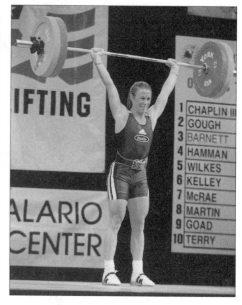

f   Recovery to a standing position.

Power Jerk

The power jerk is sometimes labeled the push jerk, which can be confusing. As we have already learned, a snatch or clean caught in a partial squat position is called a "power" snatch or clean. It makes sense that a jerk in which the body is lowered to a partial squat position, instead of a split position, should be called a power jerk.

Some lifters execute a power jerk rather than a split jerk in competition, which is within the rules. The primary rule in the jerk is that the lifter must lift the bar immediately to straight arms, without any "press out," or "muscling up" of the barbell. Lifters who power jerk in competition inevitably can split jerk (without doing a clean, but taking the bar from a rack) much more weight than they can clean. Only lifters who are confident of their ability to successfully power jerk any weight they clean should use this somewhat more precarious style.

The power jerk is an excellent assistance exercise for training the split jerk, with its emphasis on a quick, powerful upward thrust, followed by pushing the body under the bar and catching the bar securely overhead. (See figure 7.2.)

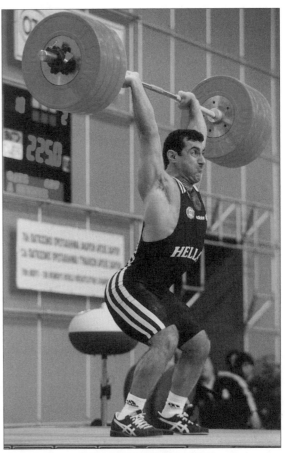

FIGURE 7.2   Akakios Kakiashvilis (GRE) uses a quick power jerk to secure the lift overhead.

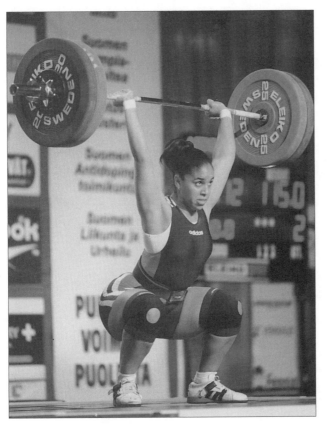

Squat Jerk

In recent years a few weightlifters have successfully performed what can only be described as a squat jerk. With little, if any, movement of the feet, this lift appears very simple to execute. Instead of stopping in a partial squat, as in the power jerk, the lifter settles into a full squat position. (See figure 7.3.) The flexibility required to get into the final receiving position is much greater than normal, and the recovery can be quite precarious. The squat jerk is not recommended for the average beginning lifter. Learn to split jerk at first; you can always experiment later with other styles.

FIGURE 7.3   Cara Heads-Lane (USA) shows great flexibility in this squat jerk.

Phases of the Jerk

Although the jerk is performed with blinding speed, you go through several stages in the process of successfully placing the bar overhead and then keeping it there until you recover to a secure position and can safely lower the weight. The explosive "power position" previously learned in the snatch and the clean is nearly identical to what you'll use in the jerk to push the bar overhead.

Starting Position

After you've successfully cleaned (squat, split, or power) the weight to your shoulders, rest momentarily with the barbell secured in the notch formed by the front part of your shoulder muscles and collarbones, without blocking your windpipe. To successfully hold the bar in this position your shoulders are protracted (moved slightly forward and upward) from their normal posture. Take several breaths to recover from the effort of cleaning the weight. Your feet remain flat and parallel to each other, about hip-width apart. Your knees and legs are straight but not rigidly locked.

Grip the bar with a closed hand, but keep your arms relaxed. Your elbows should point outward about 45 degrees from a straight-ahead orientation and should be located about halfway between perpendicular and parallel to the floor. Your eyes should be directed slightly upward, and your chin should be pulled back slightly (figure 7.1a).

Dip

With your balance in the center part of your foot, hold your last inhalation and "dip" about four to six inches. This is accomplished by flexion of the ankle, knee, and hip joints. Be sure to keep your torso straight and perpendicular to the ground. The dip is performed in a controlled manner, so the bar remains comfortably seated in its cradled position (figure 7.1b). Novices often tense their upper arms and dip so quickly that the bar is momentarily off their shoulders. When they then reverse direction and begin to jump upward, the bar drops onto their collarbones. Such an uncoordinated effort nearly always spells failure for the jerk.

You should perform the dip briskly but with the bar solidly in place. After a short dip, halt your descent (this is called the "braking phase") and rapidly transfer this eccentric muscle action in the quadriceps into a concentric muscle action, exploding upward in a vertical jump. This is another example of the plyometric effect of weightlifting exercises that can greatly aid training for performance in other sports.

Drive and Split

To perform the drive and split, you use the same triple extension of the ankles, knees, and hips used in the power position of the snatch and clean. As you rise on your toes, drive the bar off your chest by elevating your shoulders (figure 7.1c). Keep your chin back as the bar passes in front of your face.

As you push the bar a few inches off your chest, initiate a split by moving one foot forward and one rearward *while the bar is moving upward* (figure 7.1d).

Choosing which foot to split forward is very individualistic, so experiment with both feet (first without any weight) and select whichever feels most comfortable. It is easiest to initially learn and perform this movement as a simple jump with your hands on your hips. Eventually progress to an empty bar or broomstick held on your collarbones.

During the split you quickly move your feet 24 to 30 inches apart. Your hips and shoulders remain in the same vertical alignment throughout the lift. As your feet hit the split position, your arms rapidly push your body under the bar. It is very important that you push your body down rather than attempting to push the bar higher (figure 7.1e). Through proprioceptive awareness that develops after much practice, you'll quickly lower yourself to a point that coincides with the successful extension of your elbows, resulting in a solid "lockout."

It takes some time to learn to split under the bar smoothly, so don't add weight too quickly. It is crucial to success that your hips and shoulders remain under the bar, moving neither forward nor backward. Imagine a rod passing through your hips from left to right. While this rod can travel up and down, it cannot move forward or backward, nor can it twist. This image will help you focus properly on hip placement during the jerk.

It is important to move your front foot out about one and a half times the length of your shoe. To check this distance, place a piece of tape on the platform and line your toes up just behind this line. Then measure one and a half lengths of your shoe and mark that spot. This is where the toes of your front foot should end up during the split. You do not have to measure your back foot. This should place your front lower leg perpendicular to the platform with your front knee flexed about 90 degrees. This leaves you in a very mobile position in case you need to move around a bit to secure the barbell.

Keep in mind that the rear foot moves a greater distance than the front foot, so it takes a bit longer to get in place. Most lifters begin moving the rear foot first, but this is not a conscious effort.

Recovery

Once you have locked the barbell securely overhead in a solid split position, recovery to a standing position is all that remains. The recommended recovery is to straighten your front knee and hip, pushing the barbell straight up while pulling your front foot back about half the distance it covered while splitting. Throughout the recovery the barbell remains directly overhead, rising in a straight line with your hips and shoulders. Your front leg is again extended, once again splitting the distance from your front foot to your rear foot. Finally, bring your rear foot forward, parallel with your front foot (figure 7.1f). Stretch upward to your maximum height and hold this position securely before lowering the weight to the platform.

Return the bar to the platform or your shoulders depending on the number of repetitions you plan to perform. We will talk elsewhere about special jerking stands that can make the lowering process easier and safer.

Learning the Jerk

Since the jerk is a relatively simple, straightforward movement that is executed quickly, you can successfully apply the "whole" method of learning, rather than the top-down method used with the snatch and the clean. Once the starting position feels comfortable, experiment with a few practice attempts at a smooth dip. As this feels comfortable, you are ready to do the whole lift. However, some experience at placing a barbell overhead through slower lifts will be helpful.

Although the jerk is largely dependent on the leg thrust, arm and shoulder strength is needed to keep the bar overhead. It is not unusual to see a lifter jerk the weight overhead, then drop the weight while attempting to get her feet back in line for the referees' down signal. What a shame to miss a lift that has been successfully executed to this point!

Not only are the following exercises a good lead-up to learning the jerk, they also are very important parts of the overall training program to promote arm and shoulder strength and development.

Press

The press lift was part of weightlifting competition until 1973. It was eliminated largely because of problems enforcing the technical rules. However, the press remains a crucial training aid for the development of strength in the deltoids and triceps, along with contributing to a stable core posture for the muscles of the trunk.

Stand before a bar on a squat or power rack. Place your hands in a pronated (overhand) grip, with the same width you'll use for the jerk. Step under the bar with both feet, supporting the bar on your collarbones and/or shoulders (figure 7.4a). Next, lift the bar from the rack and take one or two steps backward (figure 7.4b and c). Your elbows should remain slightly in front of the bar. Take a breath, partially hold it, and straighten your elbows by pressing the bar straight up until the bar reaches arms' length (figure 7.4d). The outside portion of your elbows should be pointed directly out to the sides, and your palms should face the ceiling. Exhale as you press the bar up, inhale as you slowly lower to the starting position, and then repeat.

Push Press

The push press is an exercise designed to overload the deltoids and triceps. Since the initial stages of the push press are identical to those of the jerk, the exercise provides an excellent opportunity to learn this part of the lift with a reasonable weight.

The bar rests in the rack as with the press. Approach and remove the bar in the same fashion as you did in the press. (See figure 7.5a on page 104.) This time, after taking in a breath, descend as in the jerk, abruptly stop (figure 7.5b), then reverse direction, reaching high on your toes and pressing the bar right in front of your face (figure 7.5c). The pressing motion must be quick; you must lock your arms as soon as possible. With light weights, you can remain on your toes until the lockout occurs (figure 7.5d). With a heavier weight, return your heels immediately to the platform while pushing strongly to lock out the bar (figure 7.5e). You must push the bar at least to the top of

FIGURE 7.4   Press

a   Position yourself under the bar in the squat rack.

b   Stand up with the weight on the shoulders.

c   Step back two to three steps to clear rack.

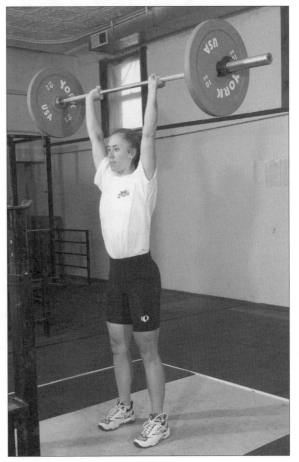

d   Press barbell overhead to arms' length.

FIGURE 7.5 **Push Press**

a   Assume the starting position.

b   Bend ankles, knees, and hips to descend.

c   Jump explosively upward and shrug shoulders.

d   Press barbell overhead with elbow extension.

e   Lock out and hold before lowering.

your head before settling back to the platform and pushing the bar overhead. Your torso remains perpendicular to the floor throughout the movement. Exhale while pressing, and then inhale as you lower the bar for the next repetition.

Power Jerk

We have previously described the power jerk. Taking the bar from a squat or power rack, the initial position is identical to that of the jerk, press, and push press (figure 7.6a). After stepping back from the rack, take a breath and dip to lower your body as in the push press (figure 7.6b). This is followed by an explosive upward jump (figure 7.6c). So far, the power jerk is no different from the push press. But, instead of pressing the bar overhead, push yourself down against the bar while flexing your ankles, knees, and hips. You'll catch the bar immediately at arms' length with no pressing action (figure 7.6d). Keep your hips and shoulders under the bar.

Once the bar is secure, straighten your ankles, knees, and hips to stand with the bar overhead (figure 7.6e). Slowly lower the bar to your shoulders and repeat the motion. Exhale while pushing up, and inhale during recovery.

The press, push press, and power jerk are exercises that should initially be performed fairly slowly while you learn the finer points of technique. It's a good idea to take a few workouts to become familiar with these movements and to be able to sharply differentiate among them before attempting any heavier weights.

Jerk

After several workouts with these lifts, you are ready to move on to the jerk. Once again, it is easiest to perform what is known as the jerk from the rack, which means you lift the bar from the squat or power rack without cleaning it. As before, step back a step or two and prepare to jerk the bar overhead. (See figure 7.7a on page 107.)

Take a breath and hold it, dip as in the push press or power jerk (figure 7.7b), apply the brakes, and explode upward. This time as the bar travels past your face, move one foot forward and the other backward (figure 7.7c). As the bar approaches the locked-out position, rapidly lower your body under the bar by straightening your elbows (figure 7.7d). If you've been successful at learning the previous exercises, the jerk should be performed effortlessly.

Lowering weights jerked overhead can eventually become a hassle and may lead to injury. At the Olympic Training Center at Colorado Springs, USA Weightlifting provides jerk "stands" for safely lowering the barbell. These consist of a large pile of plywood or particle board with a few sheets of plywood on top. This adjustable system is located just under the point to which you dip in the jerk; thus, you do not contact the stands. The barbell is lowered (after either a successful lift or a failure) and allowed to land solidly on the stands. When you are lifting heavy weights, this is an excellent way to avoid having to lower the barbell to your shoulders before performing another repetition.

FIGURE 7.6   Power Jerk

a   Assume the starting position.

b   Bend ankles, knees, and hips to descend.

c   Jump explosively upward and shrug shoulders.

d   Push body under rising bar until elbows lock out.

e   Stand with weight overhead, then lower to chest or platform.

FIGURE 7.7　Jerk

a　Assume the starting position.

b　Bend ankles, knees, and hips to descend.

c　Jump explosively upward and shrug shoulders.

d　Split feet while pushing against bar.

e　Catch bar at arms' length.

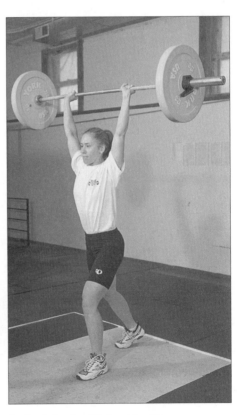

f　Push back with front foot to recover.

Jerk Behind the Neck

Although not often used in present-day training, the jerk behind the neck is a very solid way to learn the jerk movement. The bar is taken from the squat or power rack as in a squat exercise. As before, step back several steps from the rack, breathe normally, then proceed to perform a split jerk as previously learned.

Many lifters can lift more from a starting position behind the neck. This may be because of the slightly higher starting position on the trapezius muscles or because the face does not get in the way. There is also the possible psychological benefit of jerking from this somewhat stronger position.

Other Exercises

Should you identify individual weaknesses, numerous other exercises can be used on a remedial basis to improve portions of the lift. These may include a dip and drive partial movement to focus on exploding upward and forcefully lifting the bar from your shoulders. Drills are also available for learning how to step under the barbell successfully. Finally, exercises can help you get used to holding heavy weights steadily overhead. However, these are all advanced exercises that are unnecessary in the initial learning stages of the jerk. Advanced exercises should be carried out only under the supervision of a highly qualified coach.

We've taken a close, comprehensive look at the snatch, clean, and jerk. In the next chapter, we'll look at assistance exercises that complement these movements.

Pulling Exercises

8

The key to continued improvement is the early establishment of adequate technique, which we've covered in the last several chapters. Some athletes learn basic technique fairly easily, while others face a long learning curve. Once you establish adequate technique in the snatch, clean, and jerk, much of your training time is devoted simply to getting stronger. This is accomplished by (1) strengthening the individual muscle groups involved, (2) practicing the actual lifts with progressively heavier weights, and (3) using even heavier weights in what are referred to as assistance exercises. With good technique, along with added strength and power, progress in explosive lifts like the snatch and clean-and-jerk can continue for many years.

Various pulling assistance exercises are used to steadily increase strength and power for the snatch and clean. In a strength/power athlete's yearly training plan different priorities are addressed at different times of the year. Part of the training plan is geared toward gaining strength, and part is focused on sharpening sport skills for an upcoming competition. For the weightlifter, the so-called preparation (strength-building) phase focuses a great deal of attention on pulling and other strengthening exercises, mostly in two to five repetition lift sets.

Athletes from sports other than weightlifting benefit from a strong focus on pulling exercises, even in the absence of full or power versions of the classic lifts. Training with these lifts allows for the power benefits of lower-body triple extension of ankle, knee, and hip joints without having to perform the complete lift. All the muscles of the lower body are stimulated by the performance of pulling assistance exercises.

In a weightlifter's competition phase (normally the four to six weeks before a major competition), priorities switch to more technique work, especially single-repetition sets. High pull movements are included, but the emphasis is on performing the actual lift as it will occur in a contest. Depending on your sport, practicing the full lifts can be beneficial as your primary sport's major event approaches. On the other hand, athletes from some sports benefit most from successfully backing off the actual lifts and even some of the more extensive training in the weight room. They sharpen sport skills and train explosive power with plyometrics and abbreviated weight room workouts. This is a great time to use explosive assistance exercises.

Snatch-Related Pulling Exercises

A number of exercises mimic the performance of the classic snatch. These may be used in lieu of, or in addition to, regular snatch training. This can be an important consideration at different times of the year. Also, athletes of particular sports (see the discussion on "overhead" sports in chapter 11) may want to make extensive use of pulling exercises, rather than using the actual classic lifts. Extremely tall athletes who experience problems with the overhead execution of the full snatch because of limb length, poor flexibility, or other considerations will find the pulling exercises, particularly those from the blocks, easy to perform and helpful.

Muscle Snatch

An exercise created some years ago was dubbed the "muscle snatch" by USA lifters. Its purpose is to reinforce the concept of pulling through completely before turning over the wrists. The muscle snatch is basically a power snatch, but you do not rebend your knees to catch the bar overhead.

The pull is initiated like a power or regular snatch (figure 8.1a), complete with the shift to the power position (figure 8.1b and c) and an explosive vertical jump (figure 8.1d). Continue the pull while on your toes, attempting to get the bar overhead before flipping your elbows and wrists under the bar (figure 8.1e). As the flip occurs, return your heels to the platform and rapidly press the bar overhead (figure 8.1f).

Because of the height to which the bar must be pulled, only very light weights are used in this exercise. The muscle snatch should not degenerate into a wide-grip power clean and wide-grip press movement. It should remain an easy, warm-up exercise used simply to get ready for the more serious exercises that follow.

FIGURE 8.1   Muscle Snatch

a   Assume strong starting position.

b   Lift off to power position.

c   Assume power position.

d   Jump explosively upward, shrug and pull the bar.

e   Flip elbows forward.

f   Press bar to arms' length.

111

FIGURE 8.2   Snatch Pull (Bent Elbows)

Snatch Pulls

Snatch pull exercises can include many varied descriptions and titles, based largely on the actual pulling action that follows the jump. For purposes of general discussion, we'll use the term *snatch pull* to describe any pull that does not include getting the bar overhead.

Snatch Pull (Bent Elbows).   The traditional version of this movement includes jumping with the barbell after arriving in the power position, then pulling the bar as high as possible (figure 8.2a through d). A pulling height

a   **Assume starting position.**

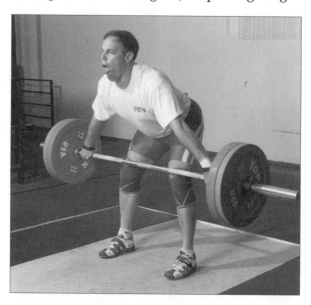

b   **Lift off to knees.**

c   **Scoop by bending ankles, knees, and hips.**

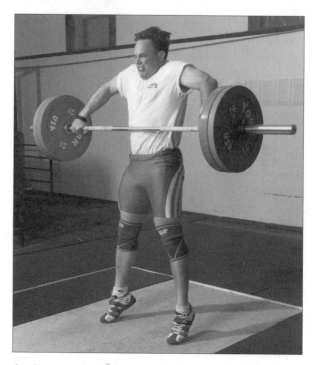

d   **Jump explosively upward, shrug, and pull bar to chest.**

approximately equal to your sternum is sought. Your elbows are kept over the bar as long as possible.

We've already mentioned the fact that you cannot possibly concentrate on hauling the bar up this high and still have time to move quickly under the bar before it begins to descend. So, many coaches recommend against performing the snatch pull with bent elbows. However, this may keep you from developing a sense of elevating your elbows beyond the point at which you shrug. Since we want your elbows to continue up while you pull under the bar, strengthening the pulling muscles in this range of motion makes sense.

Another version of this exercise involves finishing the pull without any rise on your toes. This requires good upper-back flexibility and keeps your focus on the actual pull rather than on the largely wasted effort of trying to balance on your toes.

Snatch Pull (Straight Elbows). Performing the snatch pull and finishing with a strong jump while elevating only your shoulders toward your ears (violent contraction of the all-important trapezius muscles of the upper back) is a popular version of this lift (figure 8.3a through d). Relatively heavy weights can be easily handled in this exercise, as the weak connections, your arms, do not play an active part.

This exercise can be difficult for beginners to perform properly. After the jump portion of the lift, the bar quickly accelerates upward, yet your elbows remain locked. Sometimes the resulting absorption of the weight causes the bar to move forward. It is very important to learn to flex your wrists at the point when the barbell reaches its maximum height. This helps absorb the upward thrust and maintains a stiff elbow, yet sharply contracted trapezius muscles.

Clean-Related Pulling Exercises

Pulling exercises to improve the clean are basically the same as those for the snatch, with a few notable exceptions. There is not an equivalent exercise to the muscle snatch, although such a movement could be used for the clean. In the clean, pulling the bar much beyond your navel is unnecessary, so attempts to elevate heavy weights beyond this level are not sport specific with respect to weightlifting.

Clean Pull

As we discussed in the snatch-related pulling exercises, a number of variations are available. The basic components remain identical, so experiment with all styles and use different forms of pulling in your workouts.

Clean Pull (Bent Elbows). The lift is pulled just like a clean, with the powerful triple extension of your ankle, knee, and hip joints to propel the barbell from the power position (figure 8.4a through d, page 115). After your trapezius muscles contract at the top of the jump, your elbows quickly flex to pull the barbell to the desired height, which does not need to be higher than your lower ribs. It is important that your elbows remain over the bar.

FIGURE 8.3 Snatch Pull (Straight Elbows)

a   Assume starting position.

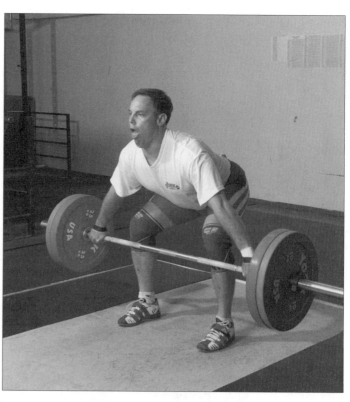

b   Lift off with knee and hip extension.

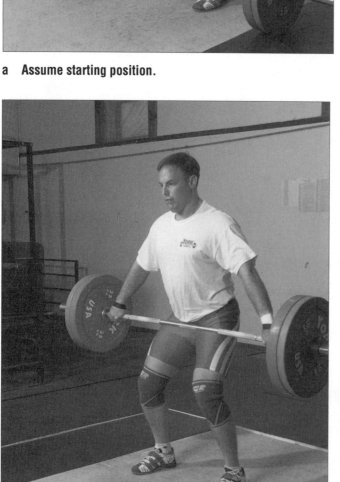

c   Scoop in to power position.

d   Jump explosively upward and shrug with arms straight.

FIGURE 8.4 Clean Pull (Bent Elbows)

a   Assume starting position.

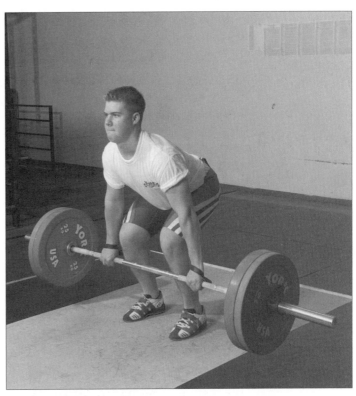

b   Lift off with knee and hip extension.

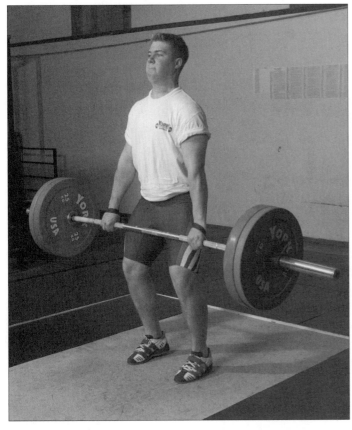

c   Scoop into power position.

d   Jump explosively upward, shrug, and pull bar to navel.

Don't focus on hauling heavy weights up much past your navel. As in the snatch pull, you should avoid pulling moderately high and dropping down to meet the bar.

Clean Pull (Straight Elbows). A clean pull with straight elbows is easy to learn and an effective alternative to performing the clean. The straight-elbow clean pull allows you to lift heavy weights explosively without the use of the weak biceps muscles. The clean pull begins just like the clean, with a strong jump from the power position, followed by a quick contraction of the trapezius muscles of your upper back, resulting in the elevation of the shoulders toward your ears (figure 8.5a through d).

Remember to flex your wrists at the top of the pull to absorb the upward momentum of the barbell.

Other Exercises

Other varieties of snatch or clean pulling exercises are available, but these are not necessary for the new lifter. First learn the lifts; then learn the basic assistance movements. Athletes who choose to specialize in weightlifting either for more strength/power benefits or as a separate sport should incorporate the following exercises into their training program.

Blocks. Performing any type of snatch or clean, or related pulls, from the blocks with the bar set in the power position can be very helpful to your lifting, but don't specialize in these lifts. Be sure to adjust either the blocks or your position to get the bar exactly where it should be. Refer to the photos in the top-down learning sequences in chapters 5 and 6 for the correct depiction of these lifts.

• **Snatch Pull From High Blocks.** Performing the snatch, power snatch, or snatch pull from the high blocks is easy and straightforward. Simply get into the power position with your balance toward the front part of your foot. Make sure your knees are over your toes. Your arms are straight, and your trapezius muscles are elongated. Your torso is inclined forward 5 to 10 degrees.

Simply explode upward in a vertical jump, remaining balanced on your toes. Either pull the bar up to midchest level or keep your elbows straight, depending on your selection of either bent- or straight-elbow pulls. Return the weights to the blocks, reset, and explosively perform the next repetition. Pulling straps are recommended.

• **Clean Pull From High Blocks.** The pull from high blocks may be done with a clean grip, but the bar starts at about midthigh level. The change in position is due to the different grip used in the two lifts. The execution of the lift is identical to the snatch version.

• **Snatch Pull From Low Blocks.** More difficult is lifting from blocks with the bar located around your knees. Since this is a difficult position even when you are in the correct position, an inch or two above or below this position may feel better, yet lead to incorrect technique. Be sure the starting position is identical to your actual lifting positions when you lift from the floor before attempting either lifts or pulls from the low blocks.

Position the bar slightly below your kneecaps, and keep your balance in the center of your foot. Your knees are nearly straight but not locked, which

FIGURE 8.5   Clean Pull (Straight Elbows)

a   Assume starting position.

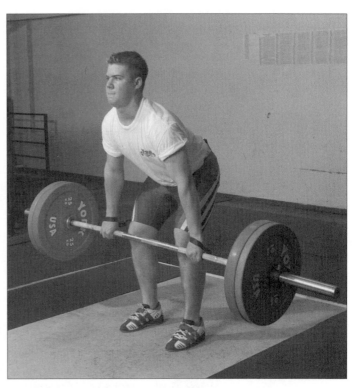

b   Lift off with knee and hip extension.

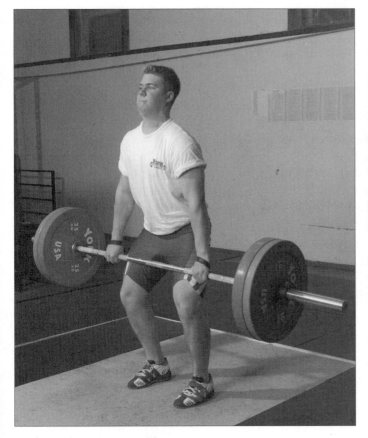

c   Scoop into power position.

d   Jump explosively upward and shrug with arms straight.

places your shoulders well in front of the bar. Your hamstrings will be in an extreme stretch at this point. Begin the lift by rapidly elevating your shoulders straight up and bringing your hips to the bar by bending your hips, knees, and ankles. This places the bar in the power position. Explode upward as you did from the high blocks. Return the weights to the blocks and repeat.

- **Clean Pull From Low Blocks.** The setup for the clean pull from low blocks is the same as that for the snatch version. Your shoulders will be a bit higher for this lift because of the difference in grip width. Lift your shoulders straight up, then bring your hips to the bar by flexing your hips, knees, and ankles. The bar will contact your legs at about midthigh level, your power position. Jump explosively upward, finishing the pull with either bent elbows or only a shrug; then return the weights to the blocks and repeat.

Elevated Pulls. Another advanced form of pulling is to stand on a small platform several inches higher than the barbell's resting surface. You then snatch, clean, or pull from this starting position. The same effect is available through the use of smaller plates if they are readily available in your gym. Since the starting position of the barbell is lower than normal relative to the shins, maintaining a neutral spine to perform the liftoff phase properly can be difficult. This type of pulling is best left for advanced lifters in need of additional variety in their training.

Deadlift. A good, strict deadlift, with a shrug at the top, can be used for either the snatch or the clean (figure 8.6a and b). Pay attention to maintaining a neutral spine in this exercise.

Partial Deadlift. A partial deadlift can be performed from the blocks or a power rack (figure 8.7a and b).

Some years ago lifters used something called a "halting deadlift" to practice strengthening the pulling motion at particular places along the pulling pathway. This isometric muscle action may provide a stimulus for an advanced weightlifter, but a beginner does not need this exercise.

While many other movements exist that can benefit your performance of weightlifting exercises, these are the basics. By focusing much of your training program on these specific pulling assistance exercises, you will gain the many benefits of training explosively for improved sport performance.

Next let's look at the other assistance exercises that are an integral part of any strength/power athlete's training regimen.

FIGURE 8.6   Deadlift

a   Deadlift start.

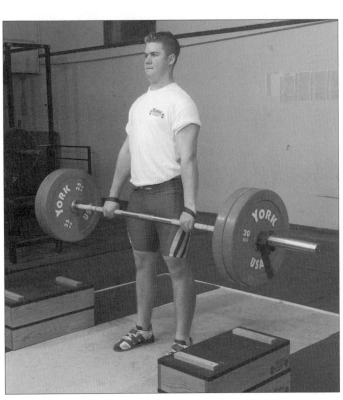

b   Deadlift midpoint.

FIGURE 8.7   Partial Deadlift

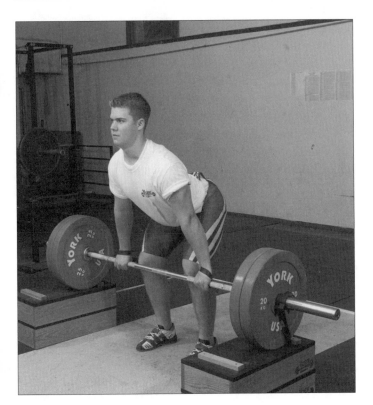

a   Partial deadlift start.

b   Partial deadlift midpoint.

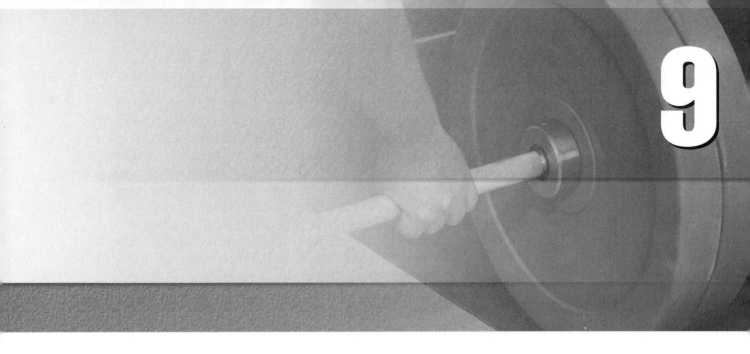

Squatting and Pressing Exercises

Two fairly distinct schools of thought exist regarding training for weightlifters. One suggests that practice should consist almost entirely of the classic lifts, along with a few supplemental pulling and squatting exercises. The second school focuses on a well-rounded development achieved mostly through the use of the classic lifts but also extensive use of other supplemental exercises to more fully prepare the body.

Since beginners bring varying levels of muscular fitness to the platform when they first learn the snatch and clean-and-jerk, some weaknesses may restrict progress. Considering the old adage You're only as strong as your weakest link, weaknesses should be eliminated in the first year of resistance training. I am a strong believer in exposing beginning weightlifters to a large variety of exercises to prepare their body completely for the heavier, more explosive work to come.

In many cases the beginning strength/power athlete should prepare through more of a bodybuilding-oriented program than a weightlifting-specific program, at least for the first 6 to 12 months. This means making use of many different exercises and developing muscles not necessarily used in weightlifting (biceps, gastrocnemius, pectorals). Multiple sets of repetitions in the 8 to 12 range are recommended. This prepares the body for the more specific work related to explosive, weightlifting-type training.

However, during the first year the neophyte lifter should drill routinely to develop excellent technique in the weightlifting-specific movements. These should be carried out only with relatively light weights to focus on speed, position, and proper execution. Properly learning the techniques associated with weightlifting exercises, plus preparing the body through a wide variety of movements, will fully prepare the body for later sport specialization. If you miss this start, you'll play catch-up for a much longer time.

Lower-Body Assistance Exercises

Most sports require a great deal of lower-body strength and power for success. Let's look at some of the basic and advanced exercises that help improve athletic performance.

Squat

The squat is an invaluable exercise in a weightlifter's training. While many varieties can be used, the basic squat is the *foundation* for not only weightlifting but also nearly every functional athletic movement in sport today.

The squat is performed with the bar resting on the upper back and shoulders. While some will refer to this as the rear squat or back squat, there really is no need for this distinction when referring to the squat.

Place the bar in a squat or power rack at about shoulder height. Grip the bar with an overhand, closed grip and step under the bar so that it rests solidly on the trapezius muscles of your upper back and your posterior deltoids. Take a breath and extend your knees and hips to stand up. Then step back two or three paces. It is always best to back away from the rack, so at the conclusion of the set you can visually spot where the bar needs to be replaced.

Place your feet flat and about shoulder-width apart, with your toes pointed either straight ahead or 10 to 15 degrees out (figure 9.1a). Take a breath; flex your ankles, knees; and hips and lower your body to a position in which the tops of your thighs are at least parallel to the floor (figure 9.1b). This lowering motion should take two to three seconds. Keep your spine straight and your chest up and look straight ahead.

Immediately reverse direction (no bouncing at the bottom) and begin the ascent. Exhale as your body works through the so-called sticking point where resistance seems the hardest. Fully extend your knees, breathe normally once or twice, and descend for the next repetition. Continue for the desired number of reps, then step back to the rack, check that the bar is located just above the bars or yokes in the squat rack, then slowly descend until the bar is securely replaced. Step away from the rack.

FIGURE 9.1   Squat

a   Squat start.

b   Squat midpoint.

Front Squat

This lift is very specific to the recovery phase of the squat clean. With the barbell resting in the rack as in the squat, grasp the bar with an overhand grip and step under the bar, placing it on your collarbones and shoulders. Maintain a full grip on the barbell; do not rest the bar on your fingertips. Stand up and take two or three steps backward (figure 9.2a).

Take a breath and descend as in the squat to a position in which the tops of your thighs are parallel to the floor (figure 9.2b). Immediately return (no

FIGURE 9.2 Front Squat

a   Front squat start.

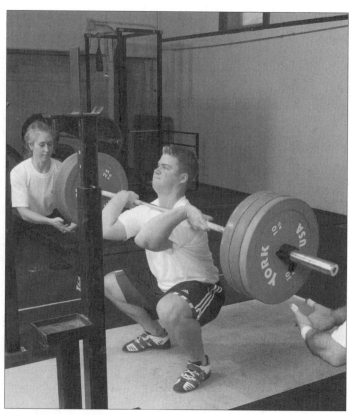

b   Front squat midpoint.

bouncing) to the standing position, exhaling while passing through the sticking point. Repeat for the desired number of repetitions; then return to the squat rack as in the squat.

Since the bar is on your shoulders rather than your back, your body may remain more erect during the front squat. This places more emphasis on the quadriceps muscles of your thighs and prevents some of the forward leaning that may occur in the squat.

Split Squat

The split squat is an advanced form of squatting that is not necessary for newcomers to weightlifting but may be useful for advanced athletes in need of specialization. Prepare a spot that includes a slightly elevated area to place your rear foot. Your rear foot rests on your toes and your sole is against a solid surface. Your front foot is securely on the floor, located just far enough in front of your rear foot to assure that your rear leg's knee intersects with your front ankle in the "down" position. Safely check and mark the proper foot placement before attempting this exercise with weight.

Get into position with either the barbell on your shoulders or a pair of dumbbells in your hands (figure 9.3a). Flex (bend) your forward ankle, knee, and hip until your rear knee lightly contacts the floor (figure 9.3b). Stand and repeat for the desired number of repetitions. Switch legs and perform the desired number of reps on the other leg. Return weights safely to their proper position.

FIGURE 9.3   Split Squat

 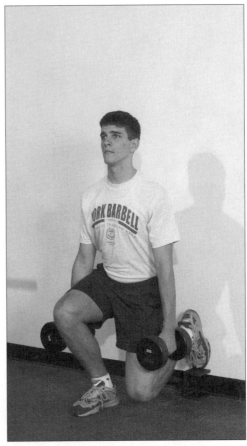

a   **Split squat start.**   b   **Split squat midpoint.**

Lunge

The lunge is very specific to those who may use the split clean. All athletes can use the lunge to strengthen their legs individually. The bar may be placed either on your upper back or on your collarbones and shoulders. Alternatively, you can use a pair of dumbbells. Be sure to try the lunge several times without any weight other than your body weight. This allows you to develop a feel for how the lunge is performed without the challenge of balancing additional weights.

Take the bar from the rack as in the squat and step back several steps (figure 9.4a). Take a breath and step forward with your right foot a distance of about 30 inches. Bend your front ankle, knee, and hip and lower your body with a forward descent until the top of your right thigh is parallel to the floor. Your left leg is supported on its toes. Your left knee is nearly straight, your hips are directly under you, and your torso is perpendicular to the floor (figure 9.4b).

Without hesitation, push upward and rearward until your right knee is nearly extended. The lunge progression may proceed in several ways. If you want to alternate legs, push upward and backward to the starting position, bringing your right foot back to its original position with a one- or two-step recovery, as in the jerk. Then step out with your left leg. Push up and back, again alternating to your opposite leg, and repeat for the desired number of repetitions.

FIGURE 9.4   Lunge

a   Lunge start.

b   Lunge midpoint.

It is also possible to push back to the starting position with your right foot, then step forward again with your right foot. Repeat the desired number of reps on your right leg; then recover and switch to your left leg.

You may also leave your right foot in place, rather than recover after each rep, and perform the assigned number of reps on your right leg first. On the last rep, recover, then switch to your left leg.

Space permitting, you may also choose to perform a "walking lunge," in which you simply move your right foot forward, recover forward to the neutral standing position, then step forward with your left leg. This sequence continues for a set distance or number of repetitions.

The dynamic lunge may be performed explosively. While in the deep split position, rapidly jump upward, reverse foot positions, and land in the lunge position with the opposite foot placement. Weight, if used, should be in the form of handheld dumbbells.

Although bodybuilders perform some other forms of lunging, none of them have the specificity of training needed for weightlifting.

FIGURE 9.5   Step-Up

Step-Up

The step-up is similar to the split squat and the lunge, but still has enough differences to make for an interesting diversion. The barbell is most conveniently located as in the squat, across your upper back and shoulders. Step back from the rack and position yourself about six inches away from a secure bench or step that allows your right thigh to be approximately parallel to the floor when your right foot is on top of the surface (figure 9.5a).

Without rocking forward or kicking off excessively with your left leg, straighten your right knee and hip until you are standing on top of the step (figure 9.5b). Bring your left foot alongside your right. There are several ways in which to continue the exercise. The easiest is to leave your left foot on top of the step and step down, placing your right foot on the floor. Then bring your left foot back to the floor. Repeat with your left leg going up first this time, followed by your right. The next repetition is right first, then left.

Alternatively, all "up" reps may be performed on one leg first, then the other leg.

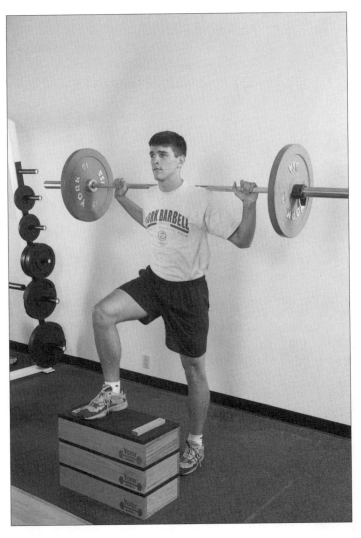

a   Step-up start.

b   Step-up midpoint.

FIGURE 9.6   Back Extension

Exercises for the Torso

The muscles of the torso connect the upper and lower body. They serve an important role in transferring power generated in "the core" to the extremities. The performance of snatch- and clean-related lifts strengthens torso muscles, but occasionally it's a good idea to throw in some other movements for variety.

Back Extension

The back extension is a very effective exercise to develop the lower back muscles. Historically called a back hyperextension, or "hyper," this exercise should never include a hyperextended spine posture. The start and finish are with your torso parallel to the floor. It can be performed on a special bench as shown in figure 9.6 or simply on an elevated surface with a training partner holding your feet in place. Regardless of the bench used, be sure to have padding under your hips or thighs.

a   **Back extension start.**

b   **Back extension midpoint.**

Once in position parallel to the floor (figure 9.6a), flex your hip joints and lower your torso toward the floor. Maintain a flat, neutral spine position as for the snatch or clean. Hands are located behind the head. Slowly descend until your torso is perpendicular to the floor, but be sure to keep the neutral spine position (figure 9.6b). Without swinging, raise back to the starting position.

To encourage a neutral spine you may need to place your hips in front of the padded area. Initially use your own body weight as resistance, slowly lowering and raising your torso for the desired number of repetitions. As you become more familiar with this exercise, gradually add weight in the form of a bar or small plate behind your head. There is no reason to use heavy weights for this exercise.

Good Morning

The good morning exercise has always been a difficult one to translate from non-English coaching manuals, not because of the nature of the exercise, but because of the name used to describe the movement. When this exercise first showed up in U.S. publications, it was known as the "bend over" exercise. Sure enough, that name wasn't going to take it very far. Some creative source concluded that since the bend at the waist (hip flexion) was similar to the motion of a gentleman bowing upon greeting a woman, this could be called the "good morning" exercise. Needless to say, editors of languages other than english never grasped this use of the lexicon, so you're more likely to see "forward bending with straight legs" or something similar when the exercise is translated.

The action, which is really hip flexion and extension while the spine remains in a neutral position, is identical to what happens with the snatch or clean, except that the barbell is not in your hands. For the good morning exercise, place the barbell on your upper back and shoulders, as in a squat. Remove the bar from the squat or power rack, step back two or three paces, and stand straight (figure 9.7a). With your toes pointed straight ahead, flex your knees just slightly and lock your spine into a neutral position with your abdominal wall contracted.

Flex your hip joints, which causes your torso to incline forward. The most sport-specific position for weightlifting is to lower your torso to a point equal to where the torso would be if the bar (when held in your hands) were just below the knees (figure 9.7b). Your balance is in the middle to rear portion of your foot, with your hips just slightly behind your heels. Avoid inclining your lower body excessively rearward. You will feel tension in your hamstrings (back of thighs).

Without hesitation, contract your gluteals and hamstrings to move your torso back to the starting position. Exhale while recovering to this posture. Repeat for the desired number of repetitions, and replace the bar in the rack.

The good morning exercise is an advanced movement. Be sure you can successfully maintain a neutral spine position before attempting this exercise. Your initial efforts should be with a dowel or empty bar.

Some sources have described performing the good morning exercise with a rounded (flexed) back, but this is not advised because of intervertebral pressure on the disks. Also, since you'll be using a neutral spine (flat back) position in all your snatch- and clean-related lifts, you'll benefit from keeping the good morning exercise sport specific.

FIGURE 9.7 Good Morning

a   Good morning start.   b   Good morning midpoint.

Some variations of this exercise include combination exercises, such as a good morning followed by a snatch-grip press behind the neck, followed by an overhead squat. Some lifters extend their hips quite rapidly, snapping back to the starting position and allowing the bar to rise from the trapezius, either in a full press behind the neck or at least a rise of six to eight inches. Note that such an exercise may cause problems when the bar returns to its starting position on the trapezius.

Stiff-Leg Deadlift

Like the good morning, the stiff-leg deadlift (SLDL) has been around for many years, evolving from a true "odd lift" to a bodybuilding exercise to a sport-specific way to train the hamstrings, hips, and lower back. As with the good morning, there are several ways in which to perform the lift, but these all involve certain risk of injury. This is an advanced exercise that requires superior flexibility and the ability to maintain a neutral spine posture.

Forward flexing of the torso should always occur with a "neutral" spine (that is, neither a flexed nor hyperextended spine). The neutral spine is crucial to success in weightlifting and in maintaining a healthy back for life. This position can be quite difficult to achieve, particularly for a novice. In fact, it is best that novices *not* perform this movement or the good morning while using any form of resistance. This is because of the advanced nature of the lift and the absolute need for safety.

FIGURE 9.8   Stiff-Leg Deadlift

Since hamstring/hip flexibility can limit your ability to get into the correct starting position, I recommend that you pick up the barbell in a conventional deadlift or clean manner. After standing, slightly flex your knees, lock your spine, and slowly bend forward at your waist by flexing your hip joints. You will feel tension in your hamstrings. Lower the bar to the floor or as far as you can without losing the neutral spine posture. After you have lowered the bar as far as you can, reverse direction and raise the barbell by hip extension back to the starting position. Repeat for the desired number of repetitions.

For those with excellent flexibility, if the correct starting position can be achieved while the barbell rests on the platform, the movement can be initiated from here (figure 9.8a through c). However, it is probably prudent to perform the lift from the top down, at least in the early learning stages.

In recent years this exercise has, for some odd reason, become known as the "Romanian deadlift" (RDL). Nicu Vlad, Olympic gold medalist weightlifter from Romania, visited and trained at the U.S. Olympic Training Center in Colorado Springs and performed SLDLs at the end of some of his workouts. Several USA lifters who were unfamiliar with the movement asked what it was. Although historically well-documented as one of four varieties of SLDL, most coaches and athletes were familiar with only the rounded-back version. Thinking a new exercise had been created, credit was given to the Romanians. Certainly neither Vlad nor the Romanians created this lift, but that's how folklore gets started.

The SLDL in its most advanced form is performed while standing on a secure riser one to four inches above the platform. This allows for a greater

a   Stiff-leg deadlift start (advanced), midpoint (basic).

b   Maintain neutral spine throughout.

c   Stiff-leg deadlift midpoint (advanced), start (basic).

131

lowering distance, thus more stress to the hamstrings. Alternatively, the lift can be performed with smaller plates, creating the same effect. The only problem today is that most plates formerly found in smaller dimensions, such as the 10-kilogram plate, now are full-size models.

Both the good morning and the SLDL have been performed with a rounded lower back and straight knees. However, due to increased intervertebral pressure and added risk of injury in this posture, neither exercise should be performed in this manner. Keep your spine neutral, just as when you snatch or clean.

Upper-Body Assistance Exercises

In the discussion and learning sequence for the jerk (chapter 7), we covered the press, the push press, and the power jerk. When the press was dropped from competition in 1973, new weightlifters did very few pressing movements. It was soon found that many weightlifters did not have the shoulder and arm strength that came from press training. This resulted in many missed jerk attempts. So, pressing is now accepted as a normal part of training regimens for competitive lifters. The press may take on any number of styles, but it is important to develop adequate pressing strength to facilitate decent jerk performance.

Press

As with the squat, the press lift is easily identified by its singular name. Confusion in the industry has led to other terms such as *military press, standing press, shoulder press, overhead press,* and others. But the bottom line remains: A press means simply pressing a weight overhead while standing.

Begin by either power cleaning the weight from the platform or taking the bar from the power or squat rack; then step back two paces. Grasp the bar with an overhand grip, using the same width grip you use to jerk. The bar should rest on your shoulders and collarbones, with your elbows pointed about 45 degrees forward and down (figure 9.9a).

Take a breath and tuck your chin; then press the bar in front of your face with a combined effort of elbow and shoulder extension. Keep the barbell close as it rises to the top of your head (figure 9.9b); then rotate your elbows to the sides and complete the elbow extension. Exhale as you press the bar upward. Take a recovery breath and slowly lower the barbell to the starting position. Repeat for the desired number of repetitions.

The press may be performed behind the neck, with varying grips, or with dumbbells, alternatively or together.

Bench Press

The bench press remains an extremely popular exercise, but it is one that can have a negative effect on weightlifting performance. Properly fixing the barbell overhead in the snatch or jerk often becomes difficult because of limited shoulder mobility resulting from increased deltoid and pectoral hypertrophy. Many powerlifters have been frustrated by this problem when trying to convert from powerlifting to weightlifting.

FIGURE 9.9   Press

a   Press start.

b   Press midpoint.

If you use the bench press as a training aid, it's a good idea to consider using a grip similar to the grip you use when performing the jerk. Press with your elbows located close to the sides of your body, minimizing the use of your pectoral muscles while still activating your triceps and deltoids.

Lie supine on a solid bench with the barbell located on uprights over your head. Always maintain a solid position on the bench, with head, shoulders, and hips firmly in contact with the surface. Keep your feet flat on the floor or on blocks or plates if the bench is too high or your legs are too short.

Always have a spotter available for bench presses. While it is not recommended to bench press without a spotter, if you do so, don't use collars on the barbell. The ability to dump weights off one end of the bar, then the other, can be a lifesaver.

Grasp the barbell with a pronated grip and lift from the supports (figure 9.10a). Pause, take in a full breath, and lower the barbell by flexing your elbows until the bar touches your chest (figure 9.10b). Then press the bar upward in a slightly arced trajectory, finishing with the bar over your face. Perform the desired number of reps and carefully replace the bar in the supports.

You may use dumbbells instead of the barbell, although this requires more effort to get the weights in place to begin the lift.

FIGURE 9.10 Bench Press

a   Bench press start.

b   Bench press midpoint.

Incline Press

The incline press was originally created by weightlifters to improve their pressing strength in the slightly laid-back fashion allowed in pressing during the 1950s and 1960s. Bodybuilders also used this exercise to stimulate muscular development in the pectoral area. Weightlifters can easily use this exercise as an adjunct to upper-body strength training.

Lie back on an incline bench with the barbell located on support racks overhead. Alternatively, place a bench without uprights under a power rack. Use a grip approximately equal to the jerk and raise the barbell off the supports (figure 9.11a). Take a breath and lower the bar to your upper chest (figure 9.11b). Upon contact, press the bar overhead via elbow and shoulder extension. The weight should travel in nearly a vertical line. Upon completion of the assigned reps, place the weight back in the racks.

You may use dumbbells instead of a barbell.

Other exercises may be used to strengthen individual muscle groups, but the exercises covered in this and the preceding chapters adequately address the majority of needs for competitive weightlifters and those looking to use weightlifting to improve other sport performance.

FIGURE 9.11   Incline Press

a   Incline press start.

b   Incline press midpoint.

10

Designing an Effective Training Program

At this stage of the book you've learned why and how explosive strength training can assist you to become a better athlete. However, it is not enough merely to use the lifts we've discussed; you must use this training wisely and correctly to assure peak performance. In this chapter you'll learn when to incorporate explosive lift training into your program.

A number of factors associated with general sport training and weightlifting-specific strength training, when properly applied, offer an increased likelihood of improved athletic results. The correct application of strength and conditioning principles in modern athletic training is a topic extensively studied by sport scientists, coaches, medical professionals, and others.

In this chapter we will focus on the basics of program planning. Program planning is not a black-and-white issue; many individual considerations must be taken into account. Although we cannot describe in great detail here the nuances of program construction for athletes of all skill levels, you'll benefit from becoming familiar with the concepts and terminology.

Many of the concepts discussed here are also relevant to your specific sport training. In today's increasingly competitive athletic arena, leaving training to random design is unwise. By adhering closely to proper training concepts, you will improve results on the field or court.

If you are fortunate enough to have a knowledgeable, highly qualified strength coach along with a well-informed sport coach to guide your training program, all you have to do is perform. However, if you serve as your own coach, awareness of the following training concepts will allow you to structure your training so that you reach your peak performance when it counts.

General Adaptation Syndrome

The basis for all modern sport training is the general adaptation syndrome, a concept strongly embraced by sport scientists and coaches as the explanation for why certain training regimens are successful. To train effectively for sport, you need to have at least a working knowledge of the design and function of the general adaptation syndrome.

The general adaptation syndrome is the creation of Hans Selye. He first wrote on the subject in the 1930s while a student in Europe. His classic text *The Stress of Life* (New York: McGraw-Hill, 1976) was first published in 1956 and serves as a primer for advanced coaching theory today. With no thought to athletic performance, Selye described general adaptation syndrome as the process by which the body responds to environmental stressors or influences that lead to change at the cellular level. Although we often consider stress a negative influence, Selye emphasized that stress is neither negative nor positive, but simply a "non-specific response of the body to any demand made upon it."

Briefly, general adaptation syndrome outlines how and why the body responds to increased demands. Provided adequate rest occurs so that cells may regenerate, changes, or adaptations, at the cellular level continue for quite some time. If proper rest is absent, the increased demands eventually lead to cellular burnout.

To understand how this all fits together, let's look at the three stages Selye identified that make up general adaptation syndrome: the alarm stage, the resistance stage, and the exhaustion stage.

Alarm Stage

During the alarm stage, the influence of a stressor causes changes to the body's response to its environment, upsetting homeostasis or cellular balance. For example, if you walk from a comfortably warm building into sub-freezing temperatures dressed in a T-shirt and shorts, your body reacts quickly to this stress by changes in posture, skin response, breathing, metabolism, and so forth.

In resistance training the alarm stage may be triggered by a new exercise; a greater (or lesser) amount of resistance; a change in the order of exercises, repetitions, or sets; a change in the rest period between sets; or similar variations. Similarly, changing any number of the variables in your specific sport will also cause a disruption in your body's sense of balance. This disruptive shock is crucial to further improvement.

When you first learn a new exercise, such as the power clean, your body experiences an alarm stage reaction, particularly if moderately heavy weights are used. The initial power clean workout or two can be fairly predictable. Your attempts may feel uncoordinated or mechanical until your body's muscular and nervous systems perform enough repetitions to elevate the barbell efficiently. The new exercise and your use of muscles not previously used may result in temporary muscle soreness, in this case, the trapezius muscles of the upper back.

Similarly, when you first report for preseason sport training, your body initially experiences an alarm stage reaction, particularly if you've not been very active physically. Such a response is temporary and normally passes within the first week of training.

Any change in training creates an alarm response. This is true even when the change is a decrease in the amount of work performed. If you suddenly switched from training six days a week to training three days a week, you would not be negatively aware of the change. But your body would most certainly be aware that things were different and respond (at the cellular level) with an alarm stage reaction. Change does not move in only one direction.

Resistance Stage

Whereas the alarm stage introduces a response to something novel, the resistance stage allows your body to shake off the change and move forward. In the resistance stage of general adaptation syndrome, your body fights back against the stressor(s) and is strengthened in its response to this outside stimulus. The stressor may be a new exercise, a heavier weight, or the introduction of sprint training. Whatever the stressor may be, your body's response to it allows you to adapt and move beyond the alarm stage.

Positive changes in your body's ability to perform the required activity are strengthened during the resistance stage. In our two previous examples, you can easily identify the process that takes place in the resistance stage. Outside in the cold, your body begins to shiver in an attempt to create movement and additional warmth. Your respiration and heart rate drop as you gradually try to acclimate to the rapid change in temperature. Your extremities begin to lose warmth, color, and circulation as your body responds with increased efforts to protect the vital organs located in the body's core.

In the weight room, after several sessions of power cleans, the trapezius muscles are no longer sore. The movement to lift the barbell to your shoulders now proceeds smoothly. You begin to apply more speed to the overall lift as you become comfortable with the movement. Your body knows what to expect, and there is no longer an alarm stage involved.

Exhaustion Stage

The exhaustion stage may occur as a result of several events. Constant alarm responses without adequate rest and recovery may cause exhaustion. On the other extreme, a failure to maintain an adequate alarm will keep your body from making further adaptations. In either case, progress comes to a standstill.

If you are exposed to the cold for a sufficiently long period of time, you may suffer from hypothermia and eventually die (the ultimate in exhaustion). In the weight room, if you constantly work at only high levels of intensity, you increase the likelihood of suffering from overtraining, or too much stress without enough rest. On the other hand, if you continue to use the same light weight you used to learn to power clean initially and do not provide your muscles with added stimulus, your body will fail to respond in a positive manner (you won't get any stronger).

You can easily see the need to maintain some sort of stress throughout the training cycle to bring your body to a higher level of performance. Your body does not make further positive changes unless it is called upon to do so. What can a coach or athlete interested in further improvement do to maintain adequate stress and make continued progress while at the same time avoid the perils of overtraining? The answer lies in what we call *periodization*.

Periodization Training

Periodization is a fancy word associated with the creation of peak athletic performance at a particular time. Periodized training provides for the manipulation of training variables, especially volume and intensity, which in turn systematically provide your body with new stressors that stimulate further progress. Proper use of periodization allows athletes to reach their peak at the right time (that is, during the most important competition).

Generally, an athlete can only hold peak condition for a couple of weeks at the most. It is extremely frustrating to reach your peak performance before or after your major competition. For athletes with a long competitive season, it is crucial to time this peak properly. For athletes who must peak to qualify for a more important competition that comes later, it is possible to peak repeatedly more than once a year, but this involves the use of miniperiodized training programs between peaks, rather than trying to remain in peak condition over a longer period of time.

Michael Stone, PhD, a widely respected sport scientist, was among the first Americans to study and publish on periodization and its application to strength training. The earliest published works on periodization and sport performance came from L.P. Matveyev of the former Soviet Union. Matveyev found that successful athletes, and weightlifters in particular, divided their training phases into off-season, preseason, and in-season cycles. Within these

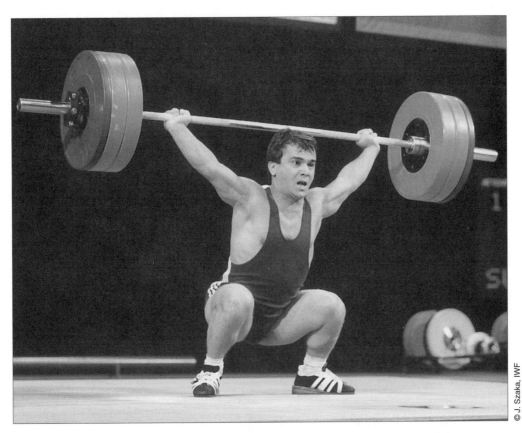

Naim Suleymanoglu (TUR), the first to win three Olympic gold medals in weightlifting, reached peak performance through periodized training.

calendar periods weightlifters further separated their training into preparation phases or competitive phases, with different volume and intensity figures associated with each.

Today's model of periodization introduces specialized terminology to refer to various phases of training:

- Macrocycle (annual plan): generally 12 months in duration
- Mesocycles (4-6 weeks): vary in purpose based on the time of the season
- Microcycle: normally refers to a one-week period

When designing a periodized training program, you will find it is easiest to start big (macro) and work backward toward small (micro). In other words, create the yearly plan and identify the most important peak first. Then, establish the various mesocycles and their specific intent (general preparation, specific preparation, or competition training). Once you know what the goal of the month, or mesocycle, is, divide that period into various weekly microcycles.

Importance of Variety

Training plans for elite athletes often appear at first glance to be randomly ordered. Weekly workouts are not identical to one another, nor are the monthly plans similar in volume or intensity. This supports the general adaptation syndrome and the need to stimulate the body to higher and higher levels of performance.

Week 1 of a preparation phase may have a different number of workouts compared to the second or third week. It is customary to set aside one week during each monthly mesocycle as an "unload" week, during which the frequency of training, along with the overall volume and intensity, drops to provide recovery from the other three weeks of training.

The primary goal of periodization is to move the athlete from general preparation consisting of high-volume, lower-intensity training in the off-season to more specific work consisting of higher-intensity, lower-volume training during the in-season. For a weightlifter, this means using somewhat lighter weights and higher repetitions during the preparation phase compared to heavier weights and fewer repetitions in the competition phase.

For the nonweightlifter, this becomes a delicate balancing act, as you need to reach a strength/power peak in resistance training (often in the off-season or preseason) before switching your priorities to conversion of this new strength to a sport-specific in-season peak. It would be impossible for an elite basketball player to reach a strength/power peak in the weight room during the basketball in-season. But reaching a strength/power peak too early or not retaining those benefits during the season makes the resistance training effort somewhat futile.

Periodization: A Must for Advanced Athletes

A great deal of specific literature is available on the subject of periodization. Although I won't cover all the details here, one important consideration deserves attention. Although periodization is required to keep an experienced athlete improving, a beginner should not be concerned with periodized training programs.

Beginners tend to make a great deal of progress regardless of how they train for a sport. This is due largely to the mastery of basic sport skills and improved physical conditioning. There is no need to manipulate training variables during the first year or so of training.

A more experienced athlete, however, should take advantage of periodized training not only in the weight room, but also for the chosen sport.

Periodized Model of Strength Training for Sports

Athletes must focus on their primary sport and be sure their abilities are sharpened to perfection to perform at their best when it is required. For a weightlifter, this might mean a state or national championship event. A football player normally peaks for maximum performance on the field in the fall. A swimmer's season usually coincides with summer months, at least for outdoor meets. Though creating and following a periodized sport training program is not difficult, athletes and their coaches are often unsure how to integrate effective resistance training into this structure.

Endurance Sports

Those who engage in long-duration, mostly aerobic sports, such as distance running, swimming, or cycling, generally fall into the category of endurance athletes. Because actual in-season sport training takes a great deal of time and energy, the same quantity and quality of effort cannot be placed on strength and power training.

With endurance athletes we normally look at the off-season as the time for general preparation work in the weight room. This is followed by increases in strength and power during the early preseason. As the competitive season approaches, resistance training shifts to an emphasis on either muscular endurance or power endurance training. The endurance athlete continues to engage in some form of in-season resistance training to maintain his gains in strength and power. Many coaches refer to this as "maintenance" training, but this is not an adequate description as we want to see actual improvements in strength and power, not just maintenance. But endurance athletes are unlikely to achieve personal bests in the weight room in-season.

Athletes from endurance sports often skip resistance training entirely during their competitive season, either because of a lack of energy or a general belief that resistance training is unnecessary in-season. Some endurance athletes believe in-season resistance training will slow them down in their events. But this is the one time when we want performance, strength, and power to remain at their highest levels. It takes a minimal amount of time and energy in-season to hold onto those hard-won gains from the off-season and preseason.

Skill Sports

Sports such as volleyball, racket sports, soccer, and the like, are often referred to as skill sports. Many skill sports include resistance training in-season. In-season workouts are reduced in frequency, as is the overall workload, but the emphasis on power remains. This sharpened power is used daily in training and regularly in competitive arenas.

Many skill sports use plyometric drills during in-season training in place of some resistance training. Athletes in sports that require explosive vertical jumps may wish to focus on plyometric training in-season, but note in the next chapter when we discuss volleyball training that plyometric training can easily overload the joints and connective tissue of players who frequently practice or play their sport. Reliance on explosive lifting and its less-intense shock to the body may be a more appropriate form of plyometric training in-season for athletes who play skill sports.

Strength and Power Sports

Sports that involve moving objects, such as football, wrestling, weightlifting, and many track and field events, rely on strength and power for success. The sport-specific training for these sports permits the continued use of weightlifting or explosive training throughout the selected sport season. Strength/power athletes often need to reach their best results in both explosive resistance training and their sport at nearly the same time.

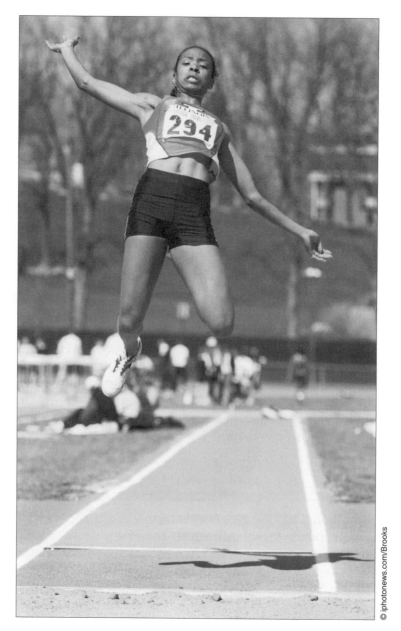

© iphotonews.com/Brooks

Attention to training variables like intensity and volume allows track and field athletes to peak when it counts.

Training Variables

You now realize that variety is important in both resistance training and in sport training. But what are some of the items that can be manipulated to provide the variety necessary to maintain progress?

A number of variables, or ingredients, in a resistance training program are frequently manipulated to coax the body along to higher and higher levels of performance. These same variables are available in your sport, but they are probably measured differently. Let's look at the most important components of a resistance training program, whether explosive or general in nature.

Volume

The term *volume* refers to how much work is performed. Volume may be recorded for a single workout, a week, a month, or the entire yearly plan. Volume can be measured in several ways, but the bottom line is that it remains a measure of the *quantity* of work.

Years ago, the sport of weightlifting commonly measured volume by tonnage, or the total amount of weight lifted, per measured cycle. This is now often referred to as *load*. To determine tonnage, you multiply the exercise weight by the number of reps per set, then multiply that figure by the number of sets performed. Add all this up, and the resulting figure is the tonnage you lifted.

To illustrate the calculation of tonnage as a measure of volume, let's compare two athletes who follow the same power clean workout, but because of unknown differences their 1-RM figures (maximum amount of weight they power clean) are much different. (See table 10.1.) The numerator is the amount of weight lifted, in this case, expressed as kilograms. The denominator is the number of repetitions lifted. The number immediately to the right of this figure is the number of sets (if more than one) performed with the same weight.

This example points out the inherent weakness when we use tonnage to measure volume. Tonnage provides useful information for an individual athlete, but it does not allow for a meaningful comparison of athletes of different abilities assigned the same training program. In this example, the tonnage for athlete A (1,100 kg) and that for athlete B (1,530 kg) are quite different. Multiply this difference by all exercises performed in a single workout, a week, a month, or even a year, and the resulting gap becomes rather wide.

If these two athletes followed the same training program, analyzing the results of their training with a comparison of volume based on tonnage would eventually prove useless. The comparison of tonnage figures to evaluate how much work a group of athletes performs becomes meaningless.

However, when we look at the *number of repetitions* performed by each athlete, we note that both athletes performed an identical amount of work.

TABLE 10.1

Power Clean

Athlete A (1-RM = 95 kg)	Athlete B (1-RM = 135 kg)
$\frac{55}{3}\ \frac{65}{3}\ \frac{75}{3}\ \frac{82.5}{2}\ \frac{87.5}{2}\ 2$	$\frac{60}{3}\ \frac{90}{3}\ \frac{110}{3}\ \frac{125}{3}\ 2$
165 + 195 + 225 + 165 + 350	180 + 270 + 330 + 750
Load or tonnage = 1,100 kg	= 1,530 kg
Repetitions performed = 15	= 15

For the past 30 or so years measuring volume by repetitions has been the favored manner for evaluating the amount of work completed. This easily allows a coach to compare the amount of work done by athletes of different body weights or gender.

Some sports relate volume to the amount of time spent training. This is not a particularly good fit for weightlifting or strength training, although it does have some application for endurance sports.

Intensity

The term *intensity* refers to the *quality* of work performed. In weightlifting and strength training, intensity is normally measured and expressed in terms of the barbell's weight (average intensity) or as a percentage of the lifter's 1-RM (relative intensity).

Average Intensity. Average intensity, normally written as Ia, is the average weight on the barbell per exercise or training period or cycle. Ia is expressed as a unit of weight, in either kilograms or pounds.

Average intensity is calculated by multiplying the weight lifted by the number of repetitions and sets performed, summing that total amount (as in the previous example's calculation of load or tonnage), and then dividing the load/tonnage figure by the total number of reps performed.

Many coaches recommend separating the intensity of the classical lifts (and their derivatives) from the intensity of squats and pulls. This is because the weights used for squats and pulls are normally greater than those handled in the lifts. Some coaches look at intensity by calculating all the exercises together.

Average intensity is a reasonable means of comparing the level of effort for an individual athlete. Since beginners tend to learn the lifts quickly and progress rapidly, it makes little sense to calculate intensity figures during the first year or so of explosive lift training. Another reason beginners do not need to be concerned with average intensity is that their early training programs consist of mostly light lifts. This renders an intensity figure without much significance. However, after the first year, average intensity calculations can be very worthwhile.

The key point to remember is that gradual increases in average intensity are critical for continued success.

Relative Intensity. Relative intensity, measured as a percentage of your maximum effort (1-RM), is expressed as a percentage rather than an absolute number, as in average intensity. A 1-RM figure is the weight you can successfully lift once, and once only. You fail to lift for one rep a slightly heavier weight, and you fail to lift for two reps a slightly lighter weight.

Most resistance training programs are designed around the 1-RM figure, so it's important to get used to talking in terms of percentages. Let's say your best power clean is 90 kilograms (about 200 pounds). In determining certain *intensity zones* around which you will train, we use the following rounded figures to represent certain percentages of your 1-RM power clean:

60%	65%	70%	75%	80%	85%	90%	95%	100%
55	57.5	62.5	67.5	72.5	77.5	80	85	90

Generally speaking, resistances below 70 percent are known as "light" intensities, those between 71 and 82 percent are "medium" intensities, those between 83 and 90 percent are considered "heavy," and those 91 percent and higher are considered "maximum" intensities. Depending on the coaching philosophy used, resistances under 50 or 60 percent (and even in some cases heavier weights) are considered "warm-up" weights and are not used to calculate intensity.

You can't lift maximum intensities every day. The lack of rest and the constant high stress loads are likely to produce an injury. The failure to allow either physical or mental recuperation may lead to symptoms of overtraining.

Likewise, training at a low intensity does not adequately stimulate the physiological changes needed to make progress. Thus, it becomes important to manipulate the intensity of your training to avoid mental or physical boredom while at the same time coaxing the body to higher performance.

Let's go back to the example used previously to illustrate volume and factor in average and relative intensity calculations. (See table 10.2.) Note that although the difference in 1-RM power cleans results in a big difference in average intensity (73.3 kg vs. 102 kg), the relative intensity figures are nearly identical (77% vs. 76%).

As with volume calculations, if a coach must compare a number of athletes with different body weight categories or skill levels or of different genders, relative intensity allows for a more meaningful comparison.

Not an Exact Science. Although coaches and scientists continue to explore meaningful ways to measure volume and intensity accurately, currently we do not have an exact science. Such numbers can be fairly easily manipulated, making some of the data highly questionable. Remember that the general principles of periodization require somewhat of a decrease in volume and somewhat of an increase in intensity for the annual plan to

TABLE 10.2

Power Clean

Athlete A (1-RM = 95 kg)	Athlete B (1-RM = 135 kg)
$\frac{55}{3}\frac{65}{3}\frac{75}{3}\frac{82.5}{2}\frac{87.5}{2}$ 2	$\frac{60}{3}\frac{90}{3}\frac{110}{3}\frac{125}{3}$ 2
165 + 195 + 225 + 165 + 350	180 + 270 + 330 + 750
Load or tonnage = 1,100 kg	= 1,530 kg
Repetitions performed = 15	= 15
Ia (average intensity) = 1,100/15, or 73.3 kg	= 1,530/15, or 102 kg
Relative intensity = 73.3/95, or 77%	= 102/135, or 76%

successfully lead to peak performance. We do need some measures of volume and intensity to accurately plan training and predict performance.

Weightlifting coaches generally agree that measuring volume as the number of repetitions performed allows for solid monitoring of progress, despite a lack of agreement on which repetitions to count. Knowledge of either your average or relative intensity is an equally valuable planning tool.

In sports such as swimming or running, intensity is often measured by speed. Recently, the advent of sophisticated heart rate monitors has allowed intensity of effort in most endurance sports to be measured by heart rate. Training is divided into the amount of time spent training in certain intensity (heart rate) zones. Although there has been some reference to heart rate as an indicator of intensity in weightlifting, you're better off getting out the calculator and figuring out the math as demonstrated earlier.

Frequency

The frequency of training refers simply to the number of workout sessions a lifter performs. This may be measured by the week, month, or year. Normal resistance training principles suggest at least three days of training most weeks, at least during the off-season and preseason phases of sport-specific training. In-season it is customary to cut resistance training to at least one day per week, although two days is preferable.

Elite weightlifters often train two or three times a day, four to six days a week. But remember, weightlifting is their chosen sport, so they do not have other distractions. Anyone using explosive training as an adjunct for their performance in another sport does not have the time or energy (or need) to be in the weight room that often.

Once again, according to the principles of the general adaptation syndrome, manipulation of your training frequency has a positive effect on progress. This is the reason behind different levels of training frequency in various stages of the annual plan.

Rest and Recovery

Rest and recovery within and between explosive lifting workouts is crucial to your success. Unlike traditional, nonexplosive resistance training, explosive lifting requires a greater intensity of effort during most lifts. If the weight is not actually heavy, you are still training power and explosive strength by attempting to move the barbell as quickly as possible. Watching elite weightlifters is an experience in seeing tremendous efforts exerted over very short periods of time. These efforts are not unlike those in other explosive events in which your immediate reaction is to catch your breath and get your heart rate back to near normal before making another similar effort.

Such effort, day in and day out, is tough on the body and requires adequate rest between sessions to allow the muscles to rebuild and grow. Add to this the fact that you have your chosen sport to train for and compete in, and you can see how important proper rest is for continued progress. Without adequate rest and recovery, you'll likely experience the exhaustion stage of the general adaptation syndrome.

Within a Workout.   The amount of time you take between sets depends largely on your present level of fitness, the relative intensity you use, some unique characteristics of your sport, and what part of the yearly plan you are in.

As with all types of training, your body will adapt to the load placed on it. But be careful in the early learning stages to allow adequate time to recover before attempting your next set. In movements such as the snatch and the clean-and-jerk, trying to perform while fatigued or not fully recovered can severely interfere with your effort. Risk of injury increases when you are not fully recovered.

When I was the USA national weightlifting coach, I was always impressed with the short periods of time between sets that were exhibited by the best European lifters backstage in a competition's warm-up area. They basically ended one set, either added weight or walked around while their seconds added the weight, then came back for their next set. Many lifters are not in good enough aerobic condition to warm up at this pace. But rather than engage in aerobic conditioning, which is pretty much a waste of time for a weightlifter, these athletes improved their functions by working out relatively nonstop.

When I coached at the Olympic Training Center, we had no chairs in the weightlifters' gym. This absence of seats kept lifters moving steadily. Among other things, it gets you through your training and out of the gym without a lot of time sitting around. This could be important in your attempts to balance specific sport training and explosive lifting.

But times do change. In recent years I have noticed when I've visited the OTC that weightlifters spend a good bit of time sitting between attempts. No doubt this helps conserve energy for the next set. Regardless of what happens between sets, weightlifters and power athletes engaged in resistance training seem to take between two and three minutes to recover between sets. This varies with the intensity used.

During in-season training, if you expect to compete with a break between efforts, as with track and field throwers and jumpers, taking a longer break between sets can prepare you for this lag in activity.

Wrestlers, by comparison, perform their resistance training fairly nonstop, which is how they compete.

Between Workouts.   The standard advice for resistance training has always been to take 48 hours between workouts to let your muscles recover and "grow." This is not bad advice, but few athletes today will make it to the top by training only Monday, Wednesday, and Friday. Don't misunderstand, there are times of the year and even times within a month when training every other day may be quite beneficial. This not only may improve recovery as in the "unload" week we covered earlier in this chapter, but the change of pace also creates a stressor that may encourage your body to make further adaptations.

Some athletes monitor either resting pulse or blood pressure to determine their readiness for the next workout. This can be important at the elite level, but for general purposes you can get by without these measurements. Do watch the quantity and quality of your sleep. Don't spend an excessive amount of time either practicing your sport or training explosively in the weight room. For beginners, the every-other-day approach, with some small amount of general fitness training on the days in between, will be adequate.

Now that you've gained exposure to some of the important variables involved in training for maximum performance, let's look at how coaches use this information. The final chapter outlines how explosive lifting is actually used in the training plans of athletes in many different types of sports.

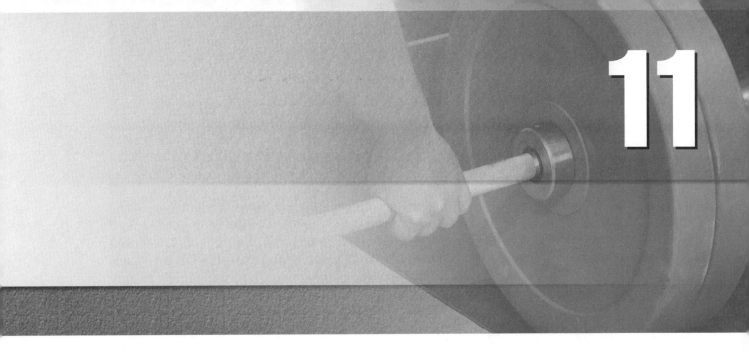

11

Sport-Specific Training Programs

An important key to improved sport performance is a well-designed sport-specific training program. This applies to both the perfection of your sport skills and the performance of additional training in the weight room. Although no amount of resistance training can take the place of mastery of specific sport skills, once sport skills are perfected, the use of systematic resistance training helps you become a stronger, more powerful athlete. In addition, perhaps the biggest benefit of resistance training is the additional protection against injury. This key consideration is often overlooked by both coaches and athletes. The ability to resist the day-to-day demands placed on your body by repeated sport practice is an important step toward continued success. Even if your sport does not require you to be larger or stronger, keep in mind that resistance training helps keep you on the playing field, and that alone is reason to get to the gym.

The use of explosive lifting exercises for improved performance in many sports is well established in the strength and conditioning profession. The key to gaining results from this form of training is your mastery of proper technique. Even if you do not have the goal of becoming a competitive weightlifter, you must strive to gain perfect technique and not just "go through the motions."

As we discussed in chapter 10, your training varies with the phase of the annual plan. This is true for both the sport-specific work on the playing field or court and the explosive resistance work done in the gym. Entire books have been devoted to the strength and conditioning aspects of many major sports. Although it is beyond the scope of this book to offer detailed training program analyses for numerous sports, this final chapter does show how explosive lifting can be successfully integrated into sport training programs.

Your specific position requirements may dictate how you use explosive lifting for improved performance. Additionally, the phase of training has an impact, as does your overall preparation for this type of advanced training. Finally, you will need qualified instruction to properly learn explosive lifting. Realize this may depend on the philosophical orientation of both your sport and strength coaches.

Many successful sport and strength and conditioning coaches enthusiastically support explosive training for their athletes. For this final chapter I contacted many such experts to seek their advice on how to integrate explosive lifting into their specific sports. The sample workouts offered here are identified as appropriate for the off-, pre-, or in-season. Keep in mind that these are just sample programs. A year-round approach to strength and conditioning requires much more detail.

BASEBALL

Baseball coaches and players have only recently accepted the concept of resistance training for improved performance. Baseball coaches have always been more accepting of speed and agility drills, but resistance training has finally earned its place in the overall picture of off-season, preseason, and in-season training.

Despite this historical reluctance toward serious resistance training, many high school, college, and professional baseball strength and conditioning coaches effectively use weightlifting-specific training for their teams. A common theme among coaches of "overhead sports" is a caution toward the use of full overhead lifts. This applies particularly to pitchers, who throw the hardest and with the greatest frequency of all position players. Despite this concern, the benefits of explosive training are easily obtained by the use of partial-pulling or pulling-only movements, as discussed in chapter 8.

Baseball players do not need to specialize in the full weightlifting movements. Partial lifts or lifts executed with dumbbells rather than a barbell are easily incorporated into the training program. Pulling exercises offer the benefits of training a total-body, multiple-joint power movement without lifting a barbell overhead.

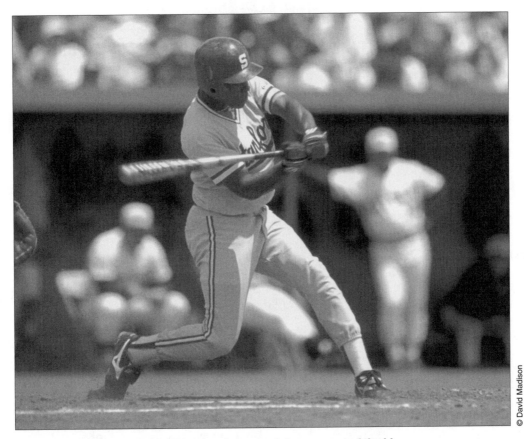

Both baseball and explosive lifting require powerful movement of the hips.

Curtis Tsuruda, assistant strength and conditioning coach at Tulane University in Louisiana, demonstrates the successful integration of explosive training for baseball players. "I've had good results (he coached LSU, the 2000 national collegiate champs) with this type of training for two reasons: (1) the lifts are performed while standing, as in playing baseball, and (2) the lifts provide a plyometric effect."

Pitchers can easily obtain both of these positive effects without performing the complete snatch movement or jerking a barbell overhead. Position players can readily benefit from performing more ballistic, total-body exercises. "I do limit the pitchers to just a few weightlifting-specific movements," says Coach Tsuruda. "This protects their shoulders against excessive use with overhead lifts. All position players use many weightlifting movements, particularly hang power cleans and clean pulls, in their off- and preseason training programs. We normally use three to six sets, with reps no higher than five."

Tsuruda, with 25 years of experience coaching baseball strength and conditioning, periodically tests his players by way of 3-RM maxes at various times of the year. He stresses excellent technique in the early stages of training and then has his athletes use both dumbbells and barbells to safely perform explosive lifts throughout the year.

Following is a sample of Coach Tsuruda's off-season LSU baseball team's resistance training program for both pitchers and position players.

153

BASEBALL

OFF-SEASON (PITCHERS)

Monday

Exercise				
DB power clean	50/5	60/4	70/3	
Clean pull	75/5	80/4	85/3	
Three-way lunge	20/8 ×3			
Good morning	40/8	50/8 ×2	60/8 ×2	
Lat pull-down	55/8	65/8	75/6	85/5 ×3
Low cable row	55/10	65/10	75/10	85/8 ×2
Pullover	Light weights 8-10 ×3			
Curl	Light weight 8-10 ×3			
Ab	Various			

Tuesday

Exercise				
Squat	50/10	60/8	70/6	80/6
Front squat	60/5	70/5	80/3	90/2
DB bench press	55/10	65/10	75/8	
Shoulder combo	Light weights			
Leg curl	Light weights			
Heel raise	Medium weights			
Triceps push-down	Medium weights			
Rotator cuff	Light weights			
Rice bucket				
Ab	Various			

OFF-SEASON (POSITION)

Monday

Exercise					
Bench press	50/10	60/8	70/8	80/6 ×3	
Shoulder combo	Medium weights 10 ×3 ea				
Squat	50/10	65/8	80/6	90/4 ×2	75/10
Glute-hamstring raise	Light weight 10-12 ×4				
Step-up	40/10 ×2	50/10 ×2			
Pullover	Medium weights 8-10 ×4				
Supine triceps press	Medium weights 10 ×4				
Forearm work	Heavy				
Rice bucket					
Shadow swing	Light				

Tuesday

Exercise					
Hang clean	50/5	60/3	70/3	80/3	85+/2 ×3
DB push press	50/6	60/5	70/3	80/3 ×4	
Clean pull	55/5	65/5	75/5	85/3	95/3 ×2
Pull-up	Bodyweight/max	Bodyweight+/max ×2			
Rotator cuff	Light weight				
DB Zottman curl	Medium weights 8-12 ×4				
Weighted bat routine					
Grip exercises (various)					
Shadow swing	Heavy				
Ab	Various				

OFF-SEASON (PITCHERS)

Thursday

Exercise	Prescription
DB power clean	as Monday
Clean pull	as Monday
Step-up	$\frac{30}{10}$ $\frac{40}{10}$ **2**
SLDL	$\frac{40}{10}$ $\frac{50}{10}$ $\frac{60}{8}$ **2**
Lat pull-down	as Monday
Low cable row	as Monday
Pullover	as Monday
Curl	as Monday
Ab	Various

Friday

Exercise	Prescription
Squat	as Tuesday
Front squat	as Tuesday
DB bench	as Tuesday
Shoulder combo	as Tuesday
Leg curl	Light weights
Heel raise	Moderate weights
Triceps kickback	Light weights
Rotator cuff	Light weights
Rice bucket	
Ab	Various

OFF-SEASON (POSITION)

Thursday

Exercise	Prescription
DB power jerk	$\frac{55}{3}$ $\frac{65}{3}$ $\frac{75}{3}$ $\frac{85}{2}$ $\frac{90+}{1}$ **3**
Jump squat	$\frac{30}{10}$ **2** $\frac{40}{10}$ **2** $\frac{50}{8}$ **2**
Three-way lunge	$\frac{20}{8}$ **3**
DB bench press	$\frac{40}{10}$ $\frac{50}{8}$ $\frac{60}{8}$ $\frac{70}{6}$ **3**
Good morning	
Shoulder combo	as Monday
Forearms	Light
Rice bucket	
Shadow swing	Light

Friday

Exercise	Prescription
Power clean	$\frac{50}{3}$ $\frac{60}{3}$ $\frac{70}{3}$ $\frac{80}{2}$ **2** $\frac{90}{2}$ **2**
DB split jerk	$\frac{55}{4}$ $\frac{65}{3}$ $\frac{75}{3}$ $\frac{85}{2}$ $\frac{90+}{1}$ **3**
Clean pull	$\frac{65}{5}$ $\frac{80}{5}$ $\frac{95}{5}$ $\frac{105}{3}$ **3**
Pull-up	as Tuesday
DB curl	as Tuesday
Rotator cuff	as Tuesday
Weighted bat	as Tuesday
Wrist roller	Medium
Grip work	(various)
Shadow swing	Heavy

Intensity-Determining Criteria

DB power clean/power clean/ clean pull/good morning/SLDL	3-RM power clean test
Push press/power jerk/jerk	3-RM DB split jerk test
Bench press	3-RM bench press test
Squat/front squat	3-RM squat test
Other exercises	Individual intensities

BASKETBALL

Basketball players benefit greatly from the proper use of explosive weightlifting exercises in their resistance training programs. The explosive nature of their sport, particularly with its emphasis on vertical power, is well suited for the classic and assistance exercises. Moreover, since basketball remains a very physical game, a stronger, more powerful player has a greater chance of surviving the long season in much better shape.

A primary concern with weightlifting training for basketball is the players' size and the possible need for modifications to get into positions to snatch or clean. Good use of partial-pulling or pulling-only movements, either from the high or low hang or blocks, may be necessary. As discussed in chapter 8, these lifts retain the positive and explosive influence of triple

© iphotonews.com/Brooks

Basketball players see the results of explosive lifting through the increase of their vertical power.

extension of the ankles, knees, and hips while avoiding possible position problems encountered by extremely tall players attempting to lift a barbell from the floor.

A strength and conditioning coach must ensure that players can properly maintain a neutral spine throughout snatch- or clean-type movements. Long before attempting to perform explosive lifts, players must demonstrate appropriate flexibility by regularly performing a stiff-leg deadlift (SLDL, see chapter 9) with an empty bar or very light weights. "This is an absolute requirement for all our players," says Al Vermeil, the successful strength and conditioning coach of the Chicago Bulls. Players who are unable to maintain a neutral spine in this movement should undergo more specific flexibility training before attempting explosive lifts. Adequate flexibility, particularly around the lower back, hips, ankles, shoulders, and wrists, is a must before attempting explosive lifting.

Coach Vermeil is a strong proponent of weightlifting movements for basketball players. "Weightlifters have an extremely high rate of force development and a great use of stored elastic energy in their muscles. Both qualities are important for speed/power sports, so this is our preferred method of lifting for basketball.

"We do a lot of lifts from the midthigh position off blocks. This forces a player to overcome inertia from zero tension, which helps develop starting strength. Some of the Bulls pull from positions below the knees, which places them in a similar position that occurs in the post. The hip extension and isometric strength of the back is very similar to that needed in low post play."

Here is how Vermeil incorporates explosive lifting into a basketball player's off-season resistance training program.

BASKETBALL

(OFF-SEASON)

- -

Monday

Power snatch/OHS	$\frac{60}{3}$				

Snatch/blocks	$\frac{60}{4}$	$\frac{70}{2}$	$\frac{80+}{2}$ **5**		

Squat	$\frac{35}{5}$	$\frac{45}{4}$	$\frac{55}{2}$	$\frac{65}{2}$	$\frac{75}{2}$	$\frac{90}{2}$

Wave squat	$\frac{30}{20}$ **2**		

Squat jump	$\frac{Bar}{4}$	$\frac{25}{4}$	$\frac{Bodyweight}{4}$ **2**

Leg curl	$\frac{Light\ weights}{8}$ **3**

Bench press	$\frac{55}{2}$	$\frac{65}{2}$	$\frac{75}{2}$	$\frac{85}{2}$	$\frac{90+}{2}$

Pull-up	$\frac{Bodyweight}{max}$ **3**

- -

Tuesday

Power clean (high hang)/ front squat	$\frac{50}{3/4}$ **2**

Box jump	4 jumps

(Blocks) Clean pulls/ clean/front squat	$\frac{65}{2/2/2}$	$\frac{75}{2/2/2}$	$\frac{80+}{2/2/2}$ **2**

Push press behind neck	$\frac{60}{2}$	$\frac{70}{2}$	$\frac{80}{2}$ **2**	$\frac{85}{2}$ **2**	$\frac{90}{2}$	$\frac{95}{2}$

One-arm cable row	8 reps, 3 sets

Back extension w/wgt	10 reps, 2 sets

- -

Wednesday

Bike/dynamic warm-up

Stretching and agility moves

Thursday

Snatch	as Monday

Speed squat $\frac{35}{3}$ $\frac{45}{2}$ $\frac{50}{1}$ **4**

Wave squat $\frac{35}{20}$ **2**

Squat jump $\frac{Bodyweight}{4}$ **4**

Box jump (12")   10 jumps, 3 sets

Pause bench press $\frac{75}{2}$ **6**

DB row $\frac{45}{8}$ **3**

Rev back extension $\frac{25}{10}$ **2**

Ab

Friday

Power clean/front squat $\frac{45}{3/4}$ **2**

Clean pull/clean (blocks) $\frac{50}{2/1}$ $\frac{60}{2/1}$ $\frac{70}{2/2}$ $\frac{80}{2/2}$ $\frac{90}{1/1}$ **2**

SLDL $\frac{60}{3}$ $\frac{80}{3}$ $\frac{90}{3}$ **3** $\frac{100}{3}$ **3**

Split squat $\frac{40}{5}$ $\frac{55}{3}$ $\frac{70}{3}$ $\frac{80}{2}$ $\frac{90}{1}$ **2**

DB press (split) $\frac{55}{5}$ $\frac{65}{4}$ $\frac{75}{3}$ **3**

Pull-down $\frac{Medium\text{-}heavy\ weight}{8\text{-}12}$ **4**

MB 400/DB back extension

Intensity-Determining Criteria

Power snatch/snatch	1-RM snatch
Power clean	1-RM power clean
Squat/wave squat/speed squat/squat jumps	1-RM squat
Front squat	1-RM front squat
Split squat	1-RM front squat
SLDL	Squat
Bench press	2-RM bench press
Push press behind neck	1-RM push press behind neck
Other exercise intensities	Individual intensities

FOOTBALL

Football was the first sport to embrace the concept of strength and conditioning for improved performance. All players benefit from the use of weightlifting exercises as part of their resistance training program, both off-season and in-season. The actual composition of a training program varies by position and individual needs.

Explosive weightlifting movements are normally placed first in the program, with the primary focus on power production. Players training under the supervision of a qualified strength coach will learn how to perform both the classic lifts and their derivatives. They will benefit from both the "power-only" (power snatch, power clean, power jerk) movements and from the full lifts. Keep in mind that because of the unique characteristics of moving an opponent's mass in more than one plane, football players also benefit from a nontraditional approach, such as the occasional use of dumbbells or one-arm lifts.

The off-season training goal for football players is to master proper technique and develop great speed of motion. The primary focus is on a quick, powerful execution of the lifts with proper resistance. Periodic testing of best performance via maximal lifts can take place in the preseason but only after players have perfected their technique in the off-season. During in-season resistance training the focus shifts to short, intense workouts designed to maximize power production.

As an example of the successful use of explosive lifts by a winning football team, let's look at how Texas A&M uses weightlifting movements. The Aggies' strength and conditioning coach, Mike Clark, says, "Football is a game that rewards powerful athletes. The use of explosive, Olympic-style weightlifting movements is the cornerstone of our program."

Football players benefit from a wide variety of lifts, increasing their power and quickness.

Coach Clark encourages his players to try many varieties of both the classic lifts and assistance exercises. He makes extensive use of combination exercises that focus on ground-based, multiple-joint movements. "We normally perform at least 75 percent of the exercises while standing, the same as when we play. Very little of our training includes seated or lying exercises, and only a few single-joint isolation movements are used."

Clark has a clear message for his players: How fast are you strong? He wants strength, but not at the expense of speed. He wants quickness, but not in the absence of strength. He seeks power, the winning formula for most sports.

Following is an example of how Coach Clark applies explosive lifting for his football players.

FOOTBALL

JUNE (PRESEASON)

Monday

Exercise	Sets/Reps
Snatch	$\frac{50}{3}$ $\frac{60}{3}$ $\frac{70}{3}$
Hang snatch	$\frac{60}{3}$ $\frac{70}{2}$ 2
Squat	$\frac{50}{10}$ $\frac{60}{8}$ $\frac{70}{6}$ $\frac{80}{6}$ $\frac{90}{3}$ 2 $\frac{70}{8}$
Lateral bound (box)	
Bench press	$\frac{50}{8}$ $\frac{60}{6}$ $\frac{70}{5}$ $\frac{80}{5}$ $\frac{80+}{3}$ 3
Lateral bound (box)	
DB row	$\frac{60}{10}$ $\frac{70}{8}$ $\frac{80}{8}$ $\frac{90}{8}$ $\frac{100}{8}$
Tempo running	8 × 100 yd (80% effort)

Tuesday

Exercise	Sets/Reps
Drop clean	$\frac{40}{5}$
Power clean	$\frac{50}{4}$ $\frac{60}{3}$ $\frac{70}{3}$ 2 $\frac{80}{3}$ 2 $\frac{90}{2}$ 2
Overhead split squat	$\frac{40}{6}$ 2 $\frac{50}{6}$ 2
DB press	$\frac{50}{10}$ $\frac{65}{8}$ $\frac{80}{6}$ $\frac{90}{6}$ $\frac{100}{5}$
Shoulder complex	
Jingle jangle	To 15 yd, back to 5 yd, back to 20 yd (40 yd) × 6 (240 yd total)

(continued on following page)

Thursday

Exercise						
Snatch	$\frac{50}{3}$	$\frac{60}{3}$	$\frac{70}{3}$	$\frac{80}{3}$	$\frac{90}{3}$	$\frac{100}{3}$
Clean pull	$\frac{75}{5}$ 2	$\frac{85}{3}$ 2	$\frac{95}{3}$ 2			
Squat	$\frac{55}{10}$	$\frac{65}{6}$	$\frac{75}{6}$	$\frac{85}{5}$	$\frac{100}{5}$	$\frac{80+}{6}$ 2
Shuffle jump						
Lateral bound						
Low incline press	$\frac{50}{10}$	$\frac{60}{8}$	$\frac{70}{6}$	$\frac{80}{5}$	$\frac{90+}{4}$	$\frac{80}{5}$ 2
One-quarter sprint	50-40-30-20-10 yd each $\times$ 2					

Friday

Exercise					
Clean-and-jerk	$\frac{50}{3/3}$	$\frac{60}{3/2}$	$\frac{70}{2/2}$	$\frac{80}{2/2}$ 2	$\frac{90+}{2/1}$ 3
Hang clean	$\frac{65}{3}$	$\frac{75}{3}$ 3			
Lunge	$\frac{40}{6/6}$	$\frac{50}{5/5}$	$\frac{60}{5/5}$ 2		
SLDL	$\frac{40}{8}$	$\frac{50}{8}$	$\frac{60}{8}$ 3		
DB bench press	$\frac{50}{10}$	$\frac{60}{6}$	$\frac{70}{6}$	$\frac{80}{6}$	$\frac{90}{6}$
Wrist roller					
Sled tow	90 lb $\times$ 20 yd $\times$ 8 reps (160 yd)				

Intensity-Determining Criteria

Snatch, hang snatch	1-RM snatch
Clean-and-jerk/power clean/ clean pull/hang clean/drop clean	1-RM clean-and-jerk
SLDL	1-RM snatch
Squat	1-RM squat
Lunge	1-RM front squat
All press movements	Appropriate 1-RM press
Overhead split squat	1-RM snatch
DB press/row	Appropriate RM in DB press/row

ICE HOCKEY

Ice hockey players use explosive weightlifting movements in addition to their other resistance training not only to improve speed and strength but also as a form of injury prevention. Over the past 15 to 20 years, strength coaches have focused on improved ice hockey performance through the use of snatch- and clean-related movements, along with the standard assistance exercises.

One of the early pioneers in the use of explosive lifting for hockey is Lorne Goldenberg, who initially worked with the Ottawa 67s and the St. Louis Blues. According to Goldenberg, "Despite early resistance from veteran players, I tested the Blues in preseason with hang power cleans. When I retested at the end of the season, the players on average had retained more than 90 percent of their performance, despite the fact they did not perform the lift during the season. This convinced me that this style of lifting is quite similar to the requirements demanded of a player."

As with the acquisition of any technical skill, Goldenberg found that drilling the basics with light weights helps to ensure that proper technique is learned. In addition, performing lifts such as a power snatch, followed by

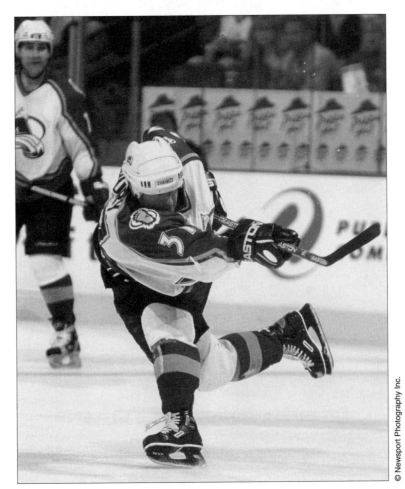

Explosive lifting pays off on the ice and helps prevent injuries.

several overhead squats, develops the core strength and stability so necessary for this style of lifting and the transmission of power to the skates.

Following is an example of a three-week off-season strength and conditioning program that Coach Goldenberg uses for one of his NHL players. Plyometric drills and sprint training occur on Wednesday and Saturday. Aerobic conditioning takes place on Tuesday and Thursday, five to six hours after the strength workout.

ICE HOCKEY

(OFF-SEASON)

Monday/Thursday

Power clean/front squat	$\frac{50}{3/3}$ $\frac{60}{3/3}$ $\frac{70}{3/3}$ $\frac{80}{2/3}$ $\frac{90}{2/2}$
Split squat (bar in front)	$\frac{60}{5}$ 2 $\frac{75}{5}$ 2
Powerskater bilateral	Highest level band, 20 reps, 3 sets
Glute-hamstring raise	6 reps, 4 sets (6-sec eccentric action)
Good morning	$\frac{40}{6}$ 2 $\frac{50}{5}$ 2 $\frac{60}{5}$ 2
Land mine bar twist	6 reps, 3 sets (explosive)
Arm catch w/single hand	6 reps, 3 sets

Tuesday/Friday

Power jerk	$\frac{50}{4}$ 2 $\frac{60}{3}$ $\frac{70}{3}$ $\frac{80}{2}$ $\frac{90}{2}$ $\frac{90+}{1}$
Atlantis side row	8 reps, 4 sets
Decline push/pull	8 reps, 4 sets
Neutral grip pull-up	Added weight, 6 reps, 4 sets
Swiss ball crunch	Added weight, 8 reps, 3 sets

Intensity-Determining Criteria

Explosive and assistance exercises are generally tested as 6-RMs, from which 1-RM estimates are established.

SOCCER

At first glance, soccer does not seem like a sport that would benefit from the elaborate strength training we've described so far. Like tennis players, soccer players are primarily interested in improved sport performance on the field. They clearly understand the benefits of agility and general conditioning drills and may even appreciate the importance of plyometric training for increased power production, but explosive lifting like the snatch or clean-and-jerk?

Strength training programs for soccer often focus more on general preparation of the body, with a heavy emphasis on the lower body and core musculature. Some coaches encourage circuit training, as this has a positive effect on the cardiorespiratory system while offering perhaps some strengthening or injury prevention.

As with all other athletes, soccer players who have not previously engaged in serious strength training should start with a program of general body preparation. At the same time they should learn the technical intricacies of explosive lifting technique with very light weights. The message is repeated: Learning technique is the first priority before moving on to heavier resistance.

© Bongarts/Martin Rose

Explosive bursts of speed and improved vertical power are required for soccer and weightlifting.

A pioneer in the area of using explosive lifting for soccer is Steve Schulz, strength and conditioning coach for the Women's United Soccer Association's 2001 national championship team, the Bay Area Cyber Rays. He also serves as strength and conditioning coach for Santa Clara University's men's soccer team in addition to Santa Clara's 2001 NCAA national champion women's soccer team. Schulz, an experienced weightlifter himself, uses the classic lifts and their derivatives to "enhance an athlete's overall training response. Most soccer players benefit from increased strength, power, balance, coordination, core strength, and improved synergistic muscular response."

Schulz has athletes use the lifts throughout the year, adjusting training based on a player's level of readiness. Once an individual demonstrates adequate strength in nonexplosive lifts, Schulz introduces the pulling motion for the snatch and the clean, in positions from the floor. "I also incorporate presses for overall upper-body strength. This soon evolves into the introduction of the push press, power jerk, and split jerk. All these lifts involve core stability, balance, and coordination." Schulz often has his athletes use dumbbells for these lifts, thereby increasing the difficulty.

Santa Clara's more advanced soccer players focus on the snatch, overhead squat, and a combination lift. A frequent combination is the squat followed immediately by a push press or power jerk. Sometimes Schulz uses a combination of a power clean, followed by a front squat, followed by a split jerk.

Goalies need to focus on more upper-body exercises, including bench and incline presses. Field players do not need this additional work but should maintain a focus on the total-body exercises.

As with other sports, soccer players should hit their peak in the weight room before the major competitions in-season. During the season, abbreviated workouts twice a week maintain the skill set and strength levels attained in the off-season and preseason. The focus on moderate loads in explosive lifts in-season ensures peak power at the most important time of the year, during the competitive season.

Let's look at an example of Coach Schulz's Santa Clara University off-season strength training for soccer.

SOCCER

Monday

Abdominal/core training

Power clean	$\frac{50}{3}$ 3	$\frac{60}{3}$	$\frac{70}{3}$ 2	$\frac{80}{3}$
Clean pull (straight arms)	$\frac{90}{3}$ 3			
Power jerk	$\frac{50}{5}$	$\frac{60}{3}$ 3	$\frac{70}{3}$ 3	
Squat	$\frac{50}{10}$	$\frac{65}{7}$	$\frac{75}{5}$ 3	
Lat pull-down	$\frac{\text{Medium weights}}{\text{8-10}}$ 3			

Quick feet drills, jump rope

Wednesday

Abdominal/core training

Hang power snatch	$\frac{50}{3}$	$\frac{60}{3}$	$\frac{70}{3}$	$\frac{80}{3}$
Snatch pull/blocks	$\frac{75}{5}$	$\frac{85}{5}$	$\frac{95}{3}$ 3	
Step-up	$\frac{45}{6}$ 2	$\frac{55}{5}$ 3		
Good morning	$\frac{40}{6}$ 2	$\frac{50}{6}$ 2		
Seated row	$\frac{\text{Medium weights}}{\text{8-10}}$ 3			

Quick feet drills, jump rope

Friday

Power clean	$\frac{55}{3}$	$\frac{65}{3}$	$\frac{75}{3}$	$\frac{85}{2}$ 2	
Clean high pulls	$\frac{95}{3}$ 3				
Squat	$\frac{60}{8}$	$\frac{70}{5}$	$\frac{80}{5}$	$\frac{90}{3}$ 2	$\frac{80+}{3}$ 2
Push press	$\frac{55}{5}$	$\frac{65}{5}$	$\frac{75}{3}$	$\frac{85}{3}$ 3	

Quick feet drills, jump rope

Intensity-Determining Criteria

Power snatch/snatch pull/good morning	1-RM power snatch
Power clean/clean pull	1-RM power clean
Power jerk/push press	3-RM power jerk
Step-up/pull-down/ab	Individual intensities

TENNIS AND RACKET SPORTS

Many racket athletes often exhibit symptoms of playing a relatively lopsided sport: (1) The dominant use of only one shoulder/arm strengthens only one side of the body and such an imbalance may lead to injury; (2) many racket athletes demonstrate a lack of overall upper-body strength; and (3) flexibility of many of the joints may be impaired because of the nature of the game.

Resistance training has a positive, balancing effect on upper- and lower-body strength, along with the core musculature. Appropriate resistance training improves power and the ability to cover ground quickly. Proper resistance training can also have a positive effect on flexibility. However, what is deemed appropriate remains a topic of debate among experts.

Because of so many cautions many coaches suggest that racket athletes train on resistance machines. Such general training may be beneficial in the early stages of development, particularly for players who are weak in many individual muscle groups. However, since the game is not played seated or lying down, this training is somewhat limited in terms of its effectiveness, and certainly does not qualify as sport-specific training.

Before attempting any free-weight strength training, and especially any explosive lifting, racket athletes must demonstrate the ability to get in the

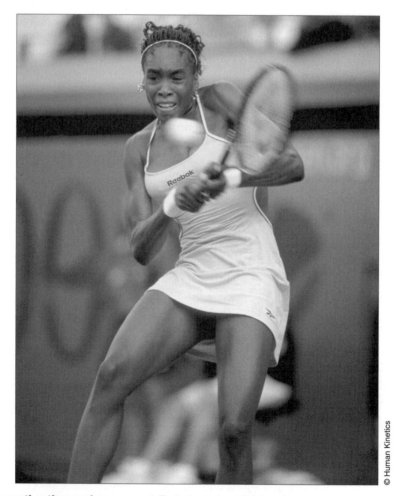

Improved reaction time and power contribute to successful tennis.

correct positions to start and complete an exercise. As with basketball players, lower back, hip, and ankle flexibility is particularly crucial.

Racket athletes may start with resistance machines, but should quickly move into free-weight exercises. After gaining overall body strength and learning proper technique, they should consider the benefits of explosive lifting for improved performance. Like coaches of players of other "overhead" sports, many tennis coaches are concerned that performing overhead lifts may be dangerous to players. But, as we saw in the example with baseball pitchers, a great deal of positive response comes from performing partial lifts that do not require overhead placement of the weight.

Clean-related lifts do not require overhead action, nor do snatch or clean high pulls. Performing these lifts improves strength and power, particularly in the lower body. As pointed out by Al Vermeil in the discussion on training basketball players, performing lifts or pulls from the hang position strengthens the core musculature. Much of tennis or racquetball is performed from a position similar to that used in starting a hang lift or high pull.

Ken Olivier, former National Association of Intercollegiate Athletics (NAIA) national tennis champion and head strength coach at the University of Texas at Tyler, is a strong proponent of resistance training for tennis players. "Weight training for tennis not only develops strength and speed, it also helps with balance. If your muscles aren't strong enough to stop on a dime, you will lose balance. No matter how good your tennis technique may be, if you can't get to the ball, you can't make the shot!"

In many cases, tennis players have little experience with free weights. Olivier cautions, "Prior experience with lifting is necessary before any advanced lifting is incorporated. Just like hitting a forehand or backhand, lifting weights is a skill to be learned."

Here is an example of how Coach Olivier incorporates explosive lifting into the off-season resistance training of his players.

TENNIS/RACKET SPORTS

Monday

Exercise	Sets/Reps
Power snatch	$\frac{40}{5}$ $\frac{50}{3}$ 2 $\frac{60}{3}$ 2
DB crossover snatch	$\frac{40}{5}$ 2 $\frac{50}{3}$ 2
Snatch high pull	$\frac{60}{5}$ $\frac{70}{5}$ $\frac{80}{5}$ $\frac{90}{3}$
Split squat	$\frac{40}{8}$ $\frac{50}{8}$ 2 $\frac{60}{6}$ 2
Lateral/forward raise	Light weights, 10-12 reps, 3 sets
Ab	Various

(continued on following page)

Wednesday

Hang power clean	$\frac{50}{5}$	$\frac{60}{3}$	$\frac{70}{3}$	$\frac{80}{2}$ **3**
Jerk from rack	$\frac{55}{3}$ **2**	$\frac{65}{3}$ **2**	$\frac{75}{2}$ **2**	$\frac{80+}{1}$ **3**
Good morning	$\frac{40}{8}$	$\frac{50}{6}$	$\frac{60}{6}$ **3**	
Lateral lunge	$\frac{20}{10}$ **2**	$\frac{30}{10}$ **2**		
DB arm curl	$\frac{50}{10}$	$\frac{60}{10}$	$\frac{70}{8}$	$\frac{80}{6}$
Rotator cuff exercises	$\frac{\text{Light weights}}{12\text{-}15}$ **3-4**			
Ab	Various			

Friday

Power clean	$\frac{55}{5}$	$\frac{65}{3}$	$\frac{75}{3}$	$\frac{85}{3}$ **3**	
Clean high pull	$\frac{75}{5}$	$\frac{85}{5}$	$\frac{95}{5}$	$\frac{105}{3}$	
Dynamic lunge	$\frac{20}{10}$	$\frac{30}{10}$	$\frac{40}{8}$ **2**		
DB bench press	$\frac{55}{10}$	$\frac{65}{10}$	$\frac{75}{8}$	$\frac{85}{6}$	$\frac{90+}{4}$
Lateral/forward raise	$\frac{\text{Light weights}}{10\text{-}12}$ **3-4**				
Lat machine pull-down	$\frac{60}{10}$	$\frac{70}{10}$	$\frac{80}{8}$	$\frac{90}{6}$ **2**	
Ab	Various				

Intensity-Determining Criteria

Power snatch/DB power snatch/ snatch pull/good morning	3-RM power snatch
Power clean/clean pull	3-RM power clean
Jerk	3-RM jerk
DB bench press	3-RM DB bench press
Split squat/lunge	5-RM leg press
DB shoulder/curl/pull-down/ab	Individual intensities

TRACK AND FIELD (ATHLETICS)

"Throwers" (shot put, discus, javelin) have embraced explosive strength training via weightlifting-specific movements for many decades. In fact, much of the training for these athletes takes place in the weight room. The explosive nature of the snatch and clean-and-jerk are specifically related to events in which a ballistic component is involved. An athlete's throwing technique continually evolves until relative stability is reached over a period of years. Early on, resistance training allows a young thrower to become more technically efficient. As technique stabilizes, resistance training becomes the primary focus of improved performance.

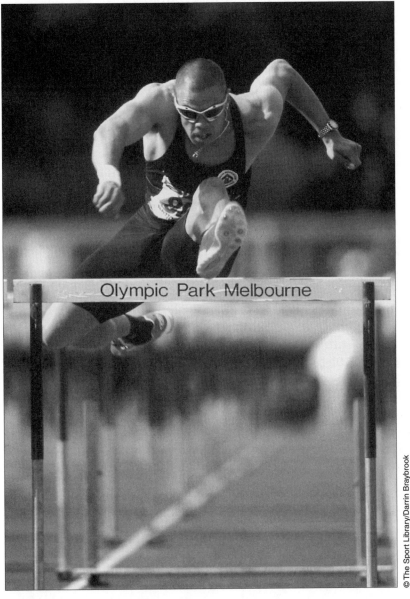

© The Sport Library/Darrin Braybrook

Track and field athletes have a great deal to gain from the snatch and clean-and-jerk because of the explosive nature of many of their events.

But what about runners and jumpers? Actually, sprinters and high/long jumpers came to accept resistance training right behind the weight throwers. Their acceptance is based partially on performance improvement and partially on injury prevention. Remaining injury-free and increasing relative strength (strength-to-weight ratio) are the keys to continued progress in track and field.

Probably the last group of athletes to accept resistance training in general, and explosive training in particular, was endurance athletes, those who run distances greater than 800 meters. However, in recent years even this group has begun to accept the wisdom of gaining strength for improved performance. Some of this relates to the physical contact that occurs in track running; some of it relates to increased time to exhaustion because of stronger muscles. Several recent studies have shown that increased resistance training has a marked effect on running economy. For example, women cross country runners at the University of New Hampshire reduced their average course times by one minute after engaging in a true strength training (not circuit training) program *in-season* with no adjustment to their running training.

One of the world's leading track and field coaches is Meg Ritchie Stone of Scotland, who made a big impact as a two-time Olympian in the discus. Stone was an early pioneer in the use of explosive training for athletics. "When I was introduced to weight training in the late '60s, the primary lifts used were the squat and the power clean. We throwers trained with weightlifters; thus we learned how to do the lifts and found our performances improved."

Stone recently served as the head coach for athletics in her native Scotland. Stone says, "I always use the snatch and clean-and-jerk for sprinters, hurdlers, jumpers, throwers, and endurance runners. The assistance movements associated with the clean are taught early on; the snatch comes later. I particularly like to use the snatch-related lifts with sprinters, javelin throwers, and jumpers."

Using a strong periodized plan, Stone manipulates athletes' intensities based on the phase of training. As many coaches have discovered, the in-season is not a time to back off on intensity. The goal of in-season resistance training is not to maintain, but to improve strength and power. However, this is also a time to focus on sport-specific skills and to avoid injury. "Particularly with sprinters in-season, I tend to go very light in some workouts and very heavy in others," Stone says.

But, the bottom line remains: All track and field athletes benefit from explosive resistance training. Here Coach Stone shares her use of explosive lifting for track and field across several different phases of the annual plan.

SPRINTERS (OFF-SEASON)

General preparation (To be used with any beginner in any event for the first 2 weeks)

Monday/Friday

Power clean (blocks)	50/5 60/5 75/5 **3**
Clean pull (floor)	50/5 60/5 75/5 **3**
SLDL	40/5 50/5 60/5 **3**
Eccentric hamstring work	
Ab	

Wednesday

Exercise	Sets
Squat	55/5 65/5 75/5 **3**
Squat/push press combo	40/5/5 60/5/5 **3**
Press behind neck	50/5 60/5 **3**
Lunge	40/5 **2** 45/5 **3**
Ab	

(During the second 4 weeks of general preparation, intensity drops to 65%, reps increase to 10, except SLDL, which remains 5 reps. In the second 4-week block the athlete returns to 5 reps and intensities are adjusted accordingly.)

Specific preparation (There are weeks when a pyramid approach is used, such as 50/5, 60/5, 70/3, 80/2.)

Monday/Friday

Exercise	Sets
Clean shrug	40/5 50/5 **3**
Clean pull (floor)	60/5 70/5 80/5 **3**
Power clean	60/5 75/5 **3**
SLDL	50/5 60/5 **3**
Eccentric hamstrings	Medium weights
Ab	

Wednesday

Exercise	Sets
Squat	50/5 60/5 70/5 80/5
Speed squat	50/3 60/3 70/3
One-quarter squat/push press combo	40/5 50/5 **2**
Walking lunge	30/5 40/5 **2**
Ab	

PRESEASON

Monday

Exercise	Sets
One-half squat	60/5 80/5 100/3 120/3 140+/3
Speed squat	50/3 60/3 70/3 80/3
Bench press	50/8 60/6 70/6 80/5 90/2-3
Dynamic lunge	Bodyweight, light weights
Ab	

Thursday

Exercise	Sets
Snatch shrug	20/5 30/3 **3**
Snatch pull (floor)	50/5 60/3 70/3 80/3 90+/3
Snatch	50/3 60/3 70/3
Snatch grip SLDL	40/5 50/3 **2**
Hamstrings	Medium weights
Ab	

(continued on following page)

TRACK AND FIELD (continued)

IN-SEASON

Monday

One-quarter squat	$\frac{50}{5}$	$\frac{80}{8}$	$\frac{110}{3}$	$\frac{140}{3}$	$\frac{160}{3}$

Explosive bench jump — Bodyweight

DB bench press — $\frac{40}{5}$ $\frac{50}{5}$ $\frac{60}{3}$ **3**

Ab

Thursday

Snatch shrug — $\frac{30}{5}$ $\frac{30}{3}$ **2**

Snatch — $\frac{30}{3}$ $\frac{40}{3}$ $\frac{50}{2}$

Dynamic lunge — Bodyweight, light weights

Hamstrings — Medium weights

Ab

Intensity-Determining Criteria

Clean/power clean/clean pull	1-RM clean
Snatch/power snatch/snatch pull/SLDL/lunge	1-RM snatch
Squat	1-RM squat
Bench press	1-RM bench press
Push press	3-RM push press
Press behind neck (PBN)	1-RM PBN

VOLLEYBALL

Early on, both indoor and outdoor ("beach") versions of volleyball embraced the benefits of explosive resistance training. Research studies have shown a positive relationship between snatch and clean-and-jerk performance and vertical jump height. The ability to forcefully and repeatedly vertical jump is a very desirable characteristic found in elite volleyball players.

However, the snatch and clean-and-jerk movements, though likely to improve jumping performance, can be overwhelming for a volleyball player with little, if any, experience in the weight room. It's crucial that players perform a periodized resistance training program throughout the year, working initially at overall body strengthening and learning the proper technique for one or more of the explosive lifts before launching into this type of training.

John Garhammer, PhD, a well-known and highly respected sport scientist who specializes in the study of biomechanics, has served as a strength coach for the volleyball and other teams at several Southern California universities. Garhammer states, "Volleyball requires an explosive vertical jump dependent on a strong, powerful lower body and the ability to quickly get your hands overhead. The snatch and clean-and-jerk lifts closely mimic what a volleyball player does in a game situation."

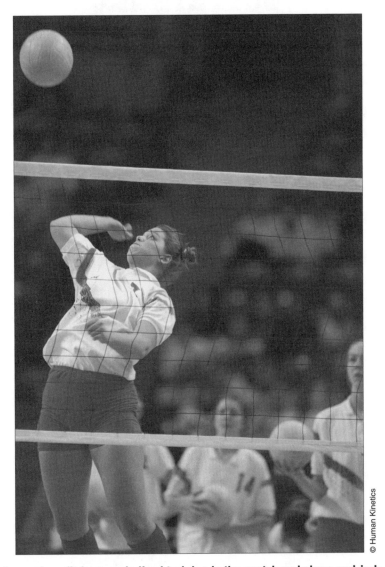

Volleyball players benefit from periodized training in the snatch and clean-and-jerk.

However, players can push beyond safe limits with a combination of volleyball practice and games, plyometric jump training, and explosive lifting movements. Garhammer cautions, "Coaches have to watch out for excessive jump training. So much stretch-shortening cycle muscle activation occurs during practice drills and games. Greater joint load forces are experienced in jump landings than in power cleans." He encourages coaches to recognize the lower impact forces of multiple-joint movements such as the squat, clean, or power jerk compared to specific jump training. Garhammer believes that explosive strength training is the best way to provide the overload needed to strengthen a player's body. His advice: Practice sport skills and get stronger through the overload provided by lifting weights. If plyometric training is used (advanced players only), it must be properly factored into a periodized training program to avoid excessive stresses to the lower body.

Here is an example of Coach Garhammer's training advice for preseason volleyball players.

VOLLEYBALL

PRESEASON (WEEK 1)

- -

Monday

Power snatch (hang)	$\frac{50}{3}$	$\frac{60}{3}$	$\frac{67}{3}$ **5**	
Snatch pull to knee	$\frac{92}{5}$ **3**			
Squat	$\frac{60}{6}$	$\frac{70}{6}$	$\frac{80}{6}$ **4**	
Bench press	$\frac{60}{6}$	$\frac{75}{6}$	$\frac{82}{6}$ **4**	
Machine row	8-12 reps, 3-4 sets			
Arm curl	8-12 reps, 3-4 sets			
Triceps press	8-12 reps, 3-4 sets			
Heel raise	12-20 reps, 4 sets			
Back extension	8-12 reps, 4 sets			
Ab	15-30 reps, 3-4 sets			

- -

Wednesday

Power jerk	$\frac{60}{3}$	$\frac{70}{3}$	$\frac{80}{3}$	$\frac{87}{3}$ **5**
Front squat	$\frac{60}{3}$	$\frac{70}{3}$ **4**		
DB incline press	8-12 reps, 3-4 sets			
Pullover	8-12 reps, 3-4 sets			
Upright row	8-12 reps, 3-4 sets			
Good morning	$\frac{\text{Light weights}}{15\text{-}30}$ **3-4**			
Ab	15-30 reps, 3-4 sets			

Friday

Power clean	$\frac{60}{3}$	$\frac{75}{3}$	$\frac{82}{3}$	**5**
Squat	$\frac{60}{3}$	$\frac{70}{3}$	$\frac{77}{3}$	**4**
Push press	$\frac{50}{3}$	$\frac{60}{3}$	$\frac{70}{3}$	**3**
DB row	8-12 reps, 3-4 sets			
Triceps press	8-12 reps, 3-4 sets			
Arm curl	8-12 reps, 3-4 sets			
Heel raise	12-20 reps, 3-4 sets			
Back extension	8-12 reps, 4 sets			
Ab	15-30 reps, 3-4 sets			

Intensity-Determining Criteria

All pulling percentages are based on best clean.
All overhead percentages are based on best power jerk.
All squat percentages are based on best squat.
Intensities for supplemental exercises are determined by individual performance, training phase, and athletic experience. Most supplemental exercises are tested at 8- to 12-RMs. Individual workout intensity on these exercises ranges from up to 10% less than the RM.

WEIGHTLIFTING

Obviously, competitive weightlifting is the sport that benefits the most from this sort of training. Athletes who choose weightlifting as their primary sport find themselves involved in a lifetime activity that offers the benefits of increased athleticism, fitness, and health. The explosive lifts are the keystone of any weightlifter's training program, although after mastering proper technique, a weightlifter spends most of his time getting stronger and more powerful.

Beyond the first few years of weightlifting training, and particularly into masters' competition (age 35 and over), the allotment of classic versus supplemental exercises shifts significantly. As with many sports, since further technique changes in the performance of the lifts are unlikely, veteran lifters don't need to spend as much time on the snatch and clean-and-jerk. More time is spent squatting and pulling, gaining additional strength and power that translates into increased performance in competition.

New weightlifters initially must spend a great deal of training time mastering technical skills. The first 6 to 12 months include a great deal of general preparation, including nonspecific bodybuilding-type exercises to promote total-body preparation. After the first year, weightlifting training settles into a periodized plan of preparation for competition.

After the initial year of training, workout composition changes about every four to six weeks. As lifters gain more experience, they must find new ways to stimulate their muscles to grow stronger and more powerful. This means different exercises, changes in repetition or set schemes, or modifications in training volume and intensity.

The preparation phase of training includes higher repetition sets with lighter weights, usually two to three reps in the classic lifts and their derivatives and three to five reps in assistance exercises such as pulls and squats. Because of this higher repetition load, the volume of training is greater here than in the competition phase. But, since the reps are higher, the intensity (average weight on the bar) is somewhat less compared to the intensity of the competition phase.

In the competition phase many of these lighter sets are eliminated, and more single efforts with higher-intensity weights are included. This manipulation of volume and intensity follows the model of periodization discussed in chapter 10.

Here is a sample workout from both preparation and competition training phases. Although it is common to train more than three days per week, especially in the preparation phase, lifters must be careful with more frequent training. The actual *amount* of training does not greatly increase; the total amount is simply spread out across more workouts. This allows the lifter to work at a high level of intensity, avoiding fatigue while maintaining adequate rest.

Mastery of the explosive lifts is the keystone to becoming a stronger and more powerful weightlifter.

WEIGHTLIFTING

PREPARATION PHASE

Monday

Power snatch $\frac{50}{3}$ $\frac{60}{3}$ $\frac{70}{3}$ $\frac{80}{2}$ **3**

Snatch $\frac{55}{3}$ $\frac{65}{3}$ $\frac{75}{2}$ $\frac{85}{2}$ $\frac{90+}{1}$ **3**

Snatch pull $\frac{75}{3}$ $\frac{85}{3}$ $\frac{95}{2}$ **2** $\frac{105}{2}$ **2**

Push press $\frac{55}{3}$ $\frac{65}{3}$ $\frac{75}{3}$ $\frac{85}{2}$ **2**

Squat $\frac{50}{6}$ $\frac{60}{5}$ $\frac{70}{4}$ $\frac{80}{4}$ $\frac{90}{3}$ **2** $\frac{75}{5}$

Wednesday

Power clean/ front squat/power jerk $\frac{50}{3/3/3}$ $\frac{60}{3/3/2}$ $\frac{70}{2/2/2}$ $\frac{80+}{2/2/1}$ **2**

Clean-and-jerk $\frac{65}{3/1}$ $\frac{75}{2/1}$ **2** $\frac{85}{2/1}$ **2** $\frac{90+}{1/1}$ **2**

Jerk from rack $\frac{65}{2}$ $\frac{80}{2}$ $\frac{90}{2}$ $\frac{100}{1}$ $\frac{105}{1}$

Clean pull $\frac{75}{5}$ $\frac{85}{3}$ $\frac{95}{3}$ $\frac{105}{2}$ **3**

Front squat $\frac{65}{3}$ $\frac{75}{3}$ $\frac{85}{3}$ **2** $\frac{90+}{2}$ **4**

Friday

Snatch $\frac{55}{3}$ $\frac{65}{3}$ $\frac{75}{3}$ $\frac{85}{2}$ $\frac{90+}{2}$ **3** $\frac{80+}{2}$ **2**

Clean-and-jerk $\frac{60}{3/2}$ $\frac{70}{3/2}$ $\frac{80}{2/2}$ **2** $\frac{90+}{2/1}$ **2**

Snatch pull (high blocks) $\frac{85}{5}$ $\frac{95}{5}$ $\frac{105}{5}$ **3**

Clean pull (low blocks) $\frac{85}{5}$ $\frac{95}{5}$ $\frac{105}{3}$ **4**

Press $\frac{50}{5}$ $\frac{60}{4}$ $\frac{70}{3}$ $\frac{80}{3}$ **3**

Squat $\frac{60}{5}$ $\frac{70}{5}$ $\frac{80}{5}$ $\frac{90}{3}$ $\frac{80}{5}$ **3**

(continued on following page)

COMPETITION PHASE

Monday

Snatch	$\frac{55}{3}$	$\frac{65}{2}$	$\frac{75}{2}$	$\frac{85}{1}$	$\frac{90+}{1}$ **3**		
Clean-and-jerk	$\frac{55}{3/3}$	$\frac{65}{2/2}$	$\frac{75}{2/1}$	$\frac{85}{1/1}$ **4**			
Snatch pull	$\frac{75}{3}$	$\frac{85}{2}$	$\frac{95}{2}$ **4**				
Push press	$\frac{55}{3}$	$\frac{65}{3}$	$\frac{75}{2}$	$\frac{85}{2}$ **2**			
Front squat	$\frac{65}{3}$	$\frac{75}{3}$	$\frac{85}{3}$	$\frac{95}{2}$ **2**	$\frac{85}{2}$	$\frac{75}{2}$	

Wednesday

Snatch	$\frac{55}{3}$	$\frac{65}{2}$	$\frac{75}{2}$	$\frac{85}{1}$ **4**	
Clean	$\frac{60}{3}$	$\frac{70}{2}$	$\frac{80}{2}$	$\frac{90+}{1}$ **3**	
Clean pull	$\frac{85}{3}$	$\frac{95}{2}$	$\frac{105}{1}$ **3**		
Press	$\frac{55}{3}$	$\frac{65}{3}$	$\frac{75}{3}$	$\frac{85}{2}$ **2**	
Squat	$\frac{60}{5}$	$\frac{70}{3}$	$\frac{80}{3}$	$\frac{85}{3}$	$\frac{90}{2}$

Friday

Snatch	$\frac{60}{3}$	$\frac{70}{2}$	$\frac{80}{2}$	$\frac{85}{1}$	$\frac{90+}{1}$
Clean-and-jerk	$\frac{55}{2/1}$	$\frac{65}{2/1}$	$\frac{75}{1/1}$	$\frac{85}{1/1}$	$\frac{90+}{1/1}$ **3**
Clean pull	$\frac{75}{3}$	$\frac{85}{2}$	$\frac{95}{1}$ **3**		
Power jerk	$\frac{65}{2}$	$\frac{75}{2}$	$\frac{85}{2}$ **3**		
Squat	$\frac{65}{3}$	$\frac{75}{3}$	$\frac{85}{3}$ **4**		

Intensity-Determining Criteria

Snatch/power snatch/snatch pull	1-RM snatch (projected)
Clean/power clean/clean pull	1-RM clean-and-jerk (projected)
Squat	1-RM squat
Front squat	1-RM front squat
Power jerk/push press	1-RM clean-and-jerk
Press	1-RM snatch

WRESTLING

Wrestling is predominantly an anaerobic sport that requires repeated explosive movements against an opponent's force. Depending on the level of competition, this effort lasts from six to nine minutes. To tolerate the high levels of lactate associated with wrestling, training must focus on speed strength and power endurance, along with technique, flexibility, core strength/stability, balance, and proprioception.

Eric Childs, strength and conditioning coach for Pennsylvania State University's wrestling team, believes strongly in the use of a periodized training program of free-weight, multiple-joint, closed-kinetic chain exercises. This includes explosive lifts, medicine ball drills, and plyometrics. "We strength train three to four days per week off-season and preseason, and two to three days per week in-season."

A solid strength training program for wrestling emphasizes increased maximum strength and improved rate of force development to produce explosive power that can be repeated over the duration of a match. "Always stress proper technique and gradual progression with your lifting program," says Childs. "Emphasize variety and make each lifting day of the week different.

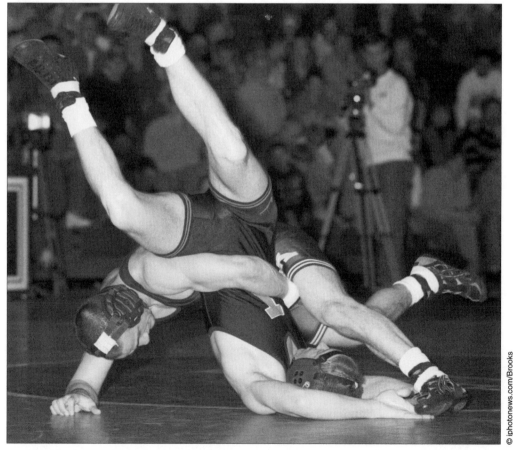

© jphotonews.com/Brooks

Wrestlers require a training program that cultivates power endurance as well as explosive movement.

"Prior to the season, we emphasize maximum strength development. But, even at this stage, we utilize complexes (a set of two different exercises) for certain body parts. The complex involves adequate recovery from one set to another, but the exercises are alternated. Also, the complex stresses a strength move followed by an explosive power move.

"During late preseason and in-season workouts, the complexes become more traditional supersets. In a superset, no recovery from one exercise to the other is given, so we work a greater emphasis on muscular endurance. The supersets allow us to fatigue the area without having to perform an excessively high number of repetitions."

Let's look at a sample of Coach Childs' use of explosive lifts for wrestlers.

WRESTLING

MAXIMUM STRENGTH PHASE

Power clean	$\frac{50}{5}$	$\frac{60}{3}$	$\frac{70}{3}$	$\frac{80}{3}$ **3**	$\frac{90+}{2}$ **2**
Push press	$\frac{55}{4}$	$\frac{65}{3}$	$\frac{75}{3}$	$\frac{85}{2}$	$\frac{90+}{1}$ **3**
Weighted pull-up	$\frac{50}{max}$	$\frac{60}{max}$	$\frac{70}{max}$	$\frac{80}{max}$	
Bench press/medball chest pass complex	$\frac{55}{8/6}$	$\frac{65}{6/5}$	$\frac{75}{5/4}$	$\frac{85}{3/3}$ **3**	
Squat/box jump complex	$\frac{55}{10/10}$	$\frac{65}{8/6}$	$\frac{75}{6/6}$	$\frac{85}{4/4}$	$\frac{90+}{1-2/2}$
Internal/external rotation	$\frac{\text{Light weights}}{10\text{-}15}$ **3**				
Four-way neck	$\frac{\text{Medium weights}}{8\text{-}12}$ **3**				

ENDURANCE CIRCUIT

2 × week

Clean/front squat/push press	$\frac{40}{5/5/3}$ **2**	$\frac{50}{4/4/3}$ **2**	$\frac{60}{3/3/3}$ **2**
DB bench press and fly (superset)	$\frac{30}{8/8}$	$\frac{40}{8/8}$	$\frac{50}{6/6}$ **3**
Rows and lat pull-down (superset)	$\frac{40}{8/8}$	$\frac{50}{8/8}$	$\frac{60}{6/6}$
Lunge (forward/lateral, superset)	$\frac{30}{6/6}$	$\frac{40}{6/6}$	$\frac{50}{6/6}$ **3**
Dip/curl superset	$\frac{30}{8/8}$	$\frac{40}{8/8}$	$\frac{50}{6/6}$ **2**
Internal/external rotation	$\frac{\text{Light weights}}{10\text{-}15}$ **3**		
Four-way neck	$\frac{\text{Medium weights}}{8\text{-}12}$ **3**		

Intensity-Determining Criteria

Power clean	2- or 3-RM
Push press	2- through 5-RM
Bench press	1-RM
Squat	1-RM

That's a quick look at how some very successful sport programs use explosive lifting to improve performance on the field or court. Each of these coaches took the time to learn the lifts and the science behind the techniques, and then work one-on-one with their athletes to ensure proper performance of the lifts. The goal of a strength and conditioning coach is to prepare players to perform at their best throughout the season. This requires a delicate balance of strength, power, flexibility, energy system fitness, speed, and agility. Explosive lifting is a great training aid for strength and conditioning coaches who know how to apply it.

Final Thoughts

Now that you have come to the end of this book, you may want to read through it again to solidify in your mind the proper lifting technique. Of course, nothing will take the place of a qualified strength and conditioning coach well versed in lifting technique to help you start on the road to explosive lifting. Also, Human Kinetics' videotape on explosive lifting will show you each exercise performed properly.

At this point you may be ready to use what you have learned in these pages to set up a strength and conditioning component to your training regimen. Be prepared to watch your sport performance improve as you master the movements used in explosive lifting. Best of luck!

Index

Note: The letters *f* and *t* after page numbers indicate figures and tables, respectively.

About the Author

Harvey S. Newton is a leading figure in the world of weightlifting. Not only is he a former U.S. Olympic team weightlifting coach and former executive director of the National Strength and Conditioning Association (NSCA), but he was also the first U.S. national coach and the first U.S. member of the International Weightlifting Federation's Scientific and Research Committee. He is the former editor in chief of NSCA's *Strength and Conditioning* and the current editor of *Strength and Health*, a publication of the York Barbell company.

Newton holds an MA in sociology from the University of Colorado. A member of the USA Weightlifting Hall of Fame, he continues to lecture nationally and internationally on strength training and weightlifting. He also serves as strength and power consultant to many sport organizations through his business, Newton Sports. Newton resides in Ormond Beach, Florida. He spends his free time lifting weights, cycling, and reading.

www.24hourteamsports.com